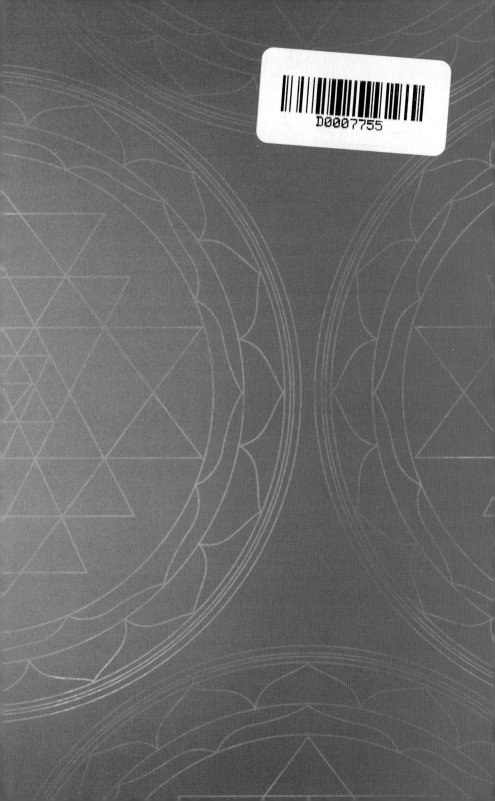

Praise for *Music and Mantras*

"I believe the book you are holding will change the world. In the years to come the inclusion of mantra practice and mindful singing into everything from yoga teacher training curricula to therapeutic treatment plans will be able to rest upon the foundation Girish has laid with this book."

—Rolf Gates, teacher and bestselling author of
Meditations from the Mat and *Meditations on Intention and Being*

"Girish has provided a pathway to an integration of personal awareness, expanded understanding, developed skill, and the experience of oneness with our Source. He invites the singer into a discipline which offers opportunities for growth, healing, and peace of mind. That wonderful mystery that while we each do our own work we are one can be seen in Girish's sharing and experienced as we join our voice with his."

—Daniel Comstock, director of
the Center for Attitudinal Healing & the Arts

"Girish has written a beautiful book with specific tools and information on this deep and life-changing practice. This book is a support to anyone finding their voice in the world."

—Mariam Gates, MEd, author of
Good Night Yoga and *Morning Yoga*

"Long before popular music was industrialized, folk music in America was focused not on the individual, but on community—people gathering together in living rooms, front porches, and town squares to play music of their ancestors and, more importantly, to sing in one voice. Girish shows how this tradition is an ancient one and why ritual is so important for nurturing wellness, not just of the individual but also among neighbors and friends. His own personal journey as a former jazz musician itself connects the dots between the West and East. Singing is as human as breathing, and this book tells us why."

—Mark Guarino, contributing music writer, *The Guardian*

"Girish is one of the rare, few integrators of the power of traditional chanting with exquisite contemporary musical artistry. For years I've found his chanting to be profoundly moving. And now with his book, *Music and Mantras*, you too can be enchanted and transformed through Girish's enlightened words and voice. This book will illuminate your mind and enhance your life with the power of mantra and chanting."

—Dan Leven, director of Leven Institute for
Expressive Movement and faculty member at Kripalu Center.

"Girish writes and sings from a nonlinear place. He journeys deep into a cave and finds the Source, the Sound, which comes up through his Heart. His book will help and inspire so many . . . as when you are blessed to hear his voice."

—Gurmukh, bestselling author and
pioneering teacher of Kundalini Yoga

"*Music & Mantras* is a beautiful contribution to all of us who seek greater harmony in our lives. It artfully combines ancient chanting with modern applications to heal our bodies and free our souls."

—Gay Hendricks, PhD, author of
The Big Leap and *Conscious Loving*

"*Music and Mantras* is a must read for all those looking to deepen their awareness of Bhakti Yoga. Girish dives into the many facets of voice, sacred pronunciation, and meanings to create a very rewarding and thorough experience for readers."

—Sridhar Silberfein, producer/
creator of Bhaktifest, producer of *River of Love*

Music and Mantras

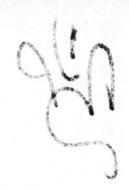

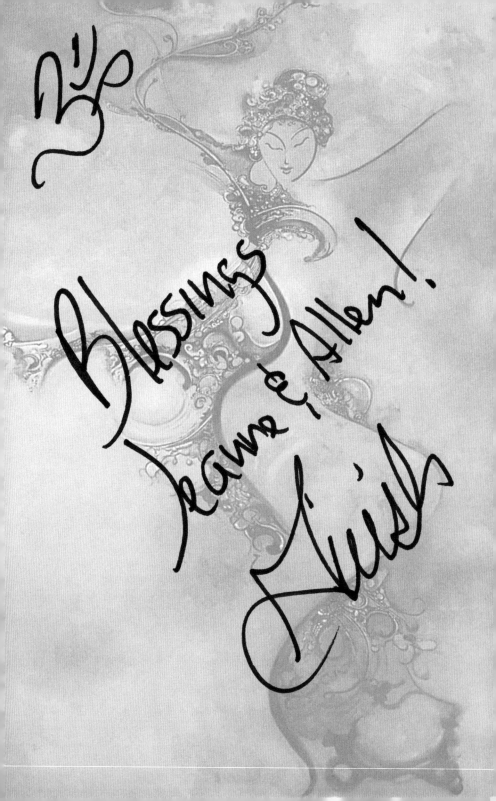

Blessings
Leanne & Allen!

Music and Mantras

THE YOGA OF MINDFUL SINGING FOR
HEALTH, HAPPINESS, PEACE & PROSPERITY

GIRISH

ATRIA

ENLIVEN BOOKS

NEW YORK   TORONTO   LONDON   SYDNEY   NEW DELHI

ENLIVEN

An Imprint of Simon & Schuster, Inc.
1230 Avenue of the Americas
New York, NY 10020

Copyright © 2016 by Mondolaya, LLC

Art by Paul Heussenstamm, Mandalas.com

First Enliven Books hardcover edition October 2016

ENLIVEN BOOKS and colophon are trademarks of Simon & Schuster, Inc.

For information about special discounts for bulk purchases, please contact Simon & Schuster Special Sales at 1-866-506-1949 or business@simonandschuster.com.

The Simon & Schuster Speakers Bureau can bring authors to your live event. For more information or to book an event, contact the Simon & Schuster Speakers Bureau at 1-866-248-3049 or visit our website at www.simonspeakers.com.

Interior design by Kyoko Watanabe

Manufactured in the United States of America

10 9 8 7 6 5 4 3 2 1

Library of Congress Cataloging-in-Publication Data has been applied for.

ISBN 978-1-5011-1220-1
ISBN 978-1-5011-1223-2 (ebook)

Contents

Contents

List of Illustrations

All artwork appearing in *Music and Mantras* is by Paul Heussenstamm.

Title page: "Blue Bali Dancer"

Foreword: "Mandala World"

Mindful Singing: "Chakra Man Gold"

The Drone Zone: "Kundalini Chakra Ladder"

Music and Mantras: "Drum Mandala"

Songbook for the Soul: "Blue Heaven Om"

Ganesh Mantras: "Ganesh"

Lakshmi Mantras: "Lakshmi in Red Poppies"

Hanuman Mantras: "Hanuman"

Shakti Mantras: "Sarasvati Space"

Shiva Mantras: "Shiva 2"

Mantras for Love, Peace, and Wisdom: "Buddha Wisdom Tree"

Conclusion: "Chakra Tree Blue"

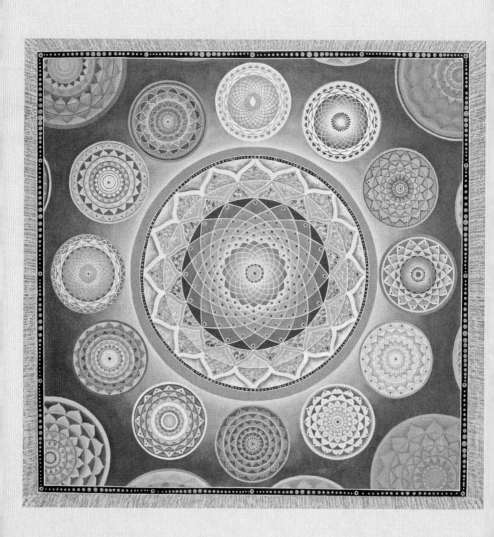

Foreword

There is a moment on the path to becoming who we are when we discover something we did not know was missing. It is often after a difficult stretch. The path has been steep and we feel that we have lost our way. But we have persisted. Suddenly there is a sense of space and light through the trees. We feel drawn to it, our steps slow, then still. We take a breath, and step out into a clearing that holds the view of the valley below, the mountains beyond, the sky above. Breathing in the beauty of the world that holds us, we experience a knowing, that is, a remembering. We stand in the presence of life's mystery and feel our place in it. We have arrived at the view from the heart. All that remains to be done is to add our sound to the larger sound.

I believe that we are here to learn: how to move, how to be still, how to love, how to be loved, when to speak up, and when to be silent. Adding our sound to the larger sound with skill and heart is something that we must learn throughout the arc of our lives. My friend Girish has given us a practice to help make this possible. Drawing from his own experience and the guidance of his teachers, Girish has put together a teaching of his own. A book that lays out how anyone who is attempting to live on purpose can bring mantra practice and mindful singing into their everyday lives.

It is no small thing to communicate both the concept of a practice and the method at the same time, and Girish has done just that. Because of this, I believe the book you are holding will change the world. I have watched one generation adopt yoga poses and in turn teach it to the next. This same possibility has been set into motion with *Music and Mantras*. In the years to come the inclusion of mantra practice and mindful singing into everything from yoga teacher training curricula to therapeutic treatment plans will be able to rest upon the foundation Girish has laid with this book. In the meantime there are the simple joys of finding our voice and giving our word.

In closing, I would like to say that I have known Girish personally for almost a decade and enjoyed his work for much longer than that. Throughout this time he has been a role model of steadfastness and devotion to his teachers, their teachings, and his practice. The disciplines he is sharing in this book he wholeheartedly embodies every day. Demonstrating with his life how the practice forms a circle, the heart stirs the voice, and the voice stirs the heart.

—Rolf Gates, teacher and author of *Meditations from the Mat* and *Meditations on Intention and Being*

Mantra Chanting is . . .

A practice that allows anyone, including non-musicians,
to experience the many life-enhancing benefits of singing.
A way for us to connect with community,
to feel a part of a vital, larger whole.
A judgement-free space,
where we can come home to ourselves.
A powerful tool for self-exploration,
self-improvement, and conscious evolution.
An elevated space where we can activate
powerful energetic archetypes that serve us in our lives.
A way for us to get out of our heads,
to be liberated from the prison of thought.
An opportunity to connect with the power
of a living tradition that stretches back for thousands of years.
A means to directly experience ourselves
as vibrational, energetic beings.

Demystifying Mantra: Basic Principles

The first time I ever remember hearing a mantra was back in 1990 when I picked up a recording of a Kundalini Yoga chant from a local bookshop in Knoxville, Tennessee. Something about the artwork on the cover of the CD and the description of the "powerful healing vibration" of the mantra spoke to me. I recall having two distinct experiences listening to that recording for the first time. One was the very visceral sense of enchantment with the vibrational quality of these sounds, the subtle thrill of opening my mind to the possibility that I was actually hearing some sort of mystical sound formula with transformational powers. Alongside my enthusiasm for this new and blissful experience, however, were the distinct protests coming from my left brain: *What the heck are these people even saying?* I couldn't make heads or tails of the words I was hearing, much less understand what they meant.

But, here's the amazing thing about this story. Just now, as I recall the experience of hearing this mantra for the first time, I can still hear the sounds and melody of this chant all these years later! Mind you, this is not a recording that became a long-term part of my music collection. I probably listened to it only a handful of times over the course of one year before moving on to other things. Somehow, in spite of the fact that I still have no actual understanding of the meaning of the mantra or even the exact words of the chant, the energetic experience of these sacred sounds is still very much alive in me. This is the inherent, magical property of mantra—the transformational energy that pulses through the vibrations of the chant. And from that first time my ears heard that CD, those healing vibrations imprinted themselves right into me, even though my conscious mind hadn't really caught up to what was happening.

As we set out on our journey to explore the yoga of mantra and chanting, we can embrace the wisdom and the grace of a beginner's mind, knowing that the mantras we chant—whether we understand exactly what they're supposed to mean or whether we're saying them exactly right—are always immensely powerful and effective. While it's true that we can refine and improve our pronunciation of these ancient sound formulas over time just as we can also deepen our understanding of the meaning and mythology these mantras contain, none of these things are prerequisites for us to have a powerful and transformative experience with chanting. This is one of the most beautiful gifts of mantra practice, really. No special skill or understanding is required. The one and only essential quality needed to enliven and empower our mantra practice is simply this: a heartfelt calling out from within.

My friend and yoga-teacher extraordinaire Janet Stone expresses this wisdom brilliantly: "Thinking that we have to have exactly the correct pronunciation of these mantras to be heard by God or the Divine is like thinking that a baby must cry in just the right way to be heard by its mother. So, first, I would say, go easy on yourself. The calling out alone is enough."

What Is Mantra?

When you hear the word *mantra*, what comes to mind? For some of us, that word might conjure up a mental image of monks clad in red and gold, swaying blissfully with eyes closed as they intone some enchanting mystical incantation. For others, the word evokes something much closer to home, firmly grounded in our own experience in practicing or at least listening to some of the world's great mantras: *Gayatri, Lokah Samasthah, Mahamrityunjaya*, or countless other Sanskrit mantras that are chanted every day by millions of people around the world.

But, if we wanted to come up with our own simple, essential definition of what a mantra really is, we could start by looking at the literal meaning of the two Sanskrit root words, *manas* and *tra*, that combine to form the word *mantra*. Looking purely at those Sanskrit roots, the word *mantra* literally means "mind tool" or "mind liberator."

Put very simply, a mantra is a sound vibration through which we mindfully focus our thoughts, our feelings, and our highest intentions. We can experience the sound vibration of mantra by singing it out loud—known as chanting—either alone or in a group; or we can experience it subtly within ourselves as we meditate on the healing energies of our chosen mantra resonating deeply within us.

Now, I'd like to point out that there's nothing in the literal meaning of the word *mantra* that suggests you have to be fluent in Sanskrit or Latin or a certain sacred language, or vow to a life of celibacy and hide out in a cave in the Himalayas. It also doesn't imply that mantra is something "exclusive," a practice meant only for a special clique of yogis and saints who know a sort of "secret" language. On the contrary, I wholeheartedly endorse mantra as one of the most inclusive and egalitarian practices out there, one that serves anyone and anywhere. And, I'll even go further to say that you don't have to join a religion—religious faith is not required to gain the benefits of mantra. You could be a Christian, Buddhist, Muslim, Catholic, or an atheist—it's not a prerequisite to learn and practice mantra. Like I said before, to enjoy the immense benefits of mantra practice, all you need to do is be present—heart and soul—with the mantra itself. The faith is in the practice.

Why Mindful Singing?

As you'll see when you begin to make your way through the pages of this book, our journey together here starts with what I hope will be an inspiring invitation: to find and express your true voice through mindful singing. Even if up to this point in your life you've been someone who would feel quite shy about opening your mouth to sing a song (unless, of course, you happened to be alone in your car or in your shower), our first bold move together will be to tell our inner Simon Cowell to take a big flying leap so that we can feel free to sing—simply for the joy of it, without judgment—to express, heal, and celebrate our unique and beautiful selves.

As we learn to open and support our singing voice in Part One of this book, we are—at the very same time—opening and expressing ourselves, literally singing ourselves more fully into being. We'll discover that our singing voice is a direct, living connection to the deepest parts of who we are, and that finding and opening that voice naturally heals, aligns, and empowers us.

By developing an awakened and powerful expression of our own voice through the practice of mindful singing, we'll have a solid foundation upon which we can begin our exploration of mantra and chanting in the later two parts of the book. There, we'll discover a rich and inspiring array of mantra practices, many of which will become powerful allies for us in our own lives as we embrace the yoga of chanting to cultivate greater health, happiness, peace, love, and wisdom.

As we'll see, certain mantras are sung out loud—or chanted— while others are experienced inside ourselves, resonating as subtle healing vibrations within our own hearts and minds; still others are written out on a page as a kind of visual meditation upon the energy of the mantra. In any and all of the ways in which we will explore mantra in the later chapters of this book, the connection with our true voice that we've awakened through mindful singing will enliven and energize our experience in powerful ways.

Basic Principles

Whether you are coming to mantra as a first-timer or a seasoned practitioner, my hope is that what you don't know or do know about this rich and beautiful practice becomes an altogether fresh and revitalized experience as you explore the chapters ahead. This book is about an inspiring new approach to mantra practice, one that links an ancient yogic tradition with the latest insights of modern science, revealing a contemporary understanding of how we can embrace the yoga of chanting to affect real, positive change in our daily lives.

Before we dive in, it's important to point out that there is a rich and long history of mantra that goes back thousands of years.

It's a tradition with a legacy that has influenced many cultures and many millions of people, one that is far too expansive for me to fully capture in this one book. However, I do want to share a little of mantra's history—to give you a taste of this perennial and evolving practice—a movement that you are now a part of.

A Little Mantra History

Human beings have been chanting mantras of countless varieties in spiritual and meditation traditions the world over for thousands and thousands of years. Consider the vintage of a mantra like the famous *Gayatri*, which hails from one of the oldest literary works known to man, India's most ancient scripture, the *Rig Veda*. Scholars peg the first written appearance of the *Gayatri* to at least three thousand years ago, although its existence as an oral tradition likely preceded that by thousands of years more. Tallying all that up, we're talking about a mantra that has been a part of the human experience for somewhere between four thousand and six thousand years. Looking back through the mists of time to merely the three-thousand-year mark still lands us squarely in a period in which the Egyptian empire was just hitting its stride with Ramses II sitting in the pharaoh's chair while the Mayan empire was still just a twinkle in Central America's eye.

Despite this mantra's almost inconceivably distant heritage, during the very same day on which you read this sentence the *Gayatri* mantra will be chanted by millions of devoted Hindus as well as other enthusiastic mantra aficionados all around the world. In fact, the practice of mantra chanting is very much alive and well today not only in India, but on every continent on earth. Although the mantras we'll explore together in this book arise from India's Hindu tradition, nearly every one of the world's other great spiritual traditions also embraces mantra and chanting practice in one form or another as a vital part of the path. Some of the most widely known examples from these other traditions include Buddhism's *Om Mani Padme Hum*, Christianity's *Ave Maria*, Judaism's *Nigun* chants, Jainism's *Namokar* mantra, Sufism's *La ilaha illAllah*, and Sikhism's *Mool Mantar*, among many others. The cultures represented by this widely diverse group of spiritual traditions span the globe, revealing the nearly universal appeal of this ancient practice.

So, we know from history that for thousands of years, human beings by the millions have turned to the practice of mantra as a means of cultivating harmony, wisdom, healing, peace, loving-kindness, personal growth, and self-discovery. Through all the seismic shifts that have transformed human culture over a vast period of time spanning from before the birth of written language during the Bronze Age in the fifteenth century BC all the way to the present day, mantra practice has been a constant staple of human life for millions of people around the globe. Why? Because it works. However, it's only now, in the twenty-first century, that we're able to pull back the curtain a little on this ancient practice to understand how and why mantra is so effective.

The book you now hold in your hands offers an opportunity to learn and experience the powerfully healing practice of mantra for yourself, to make it an inspiring and empowering part of your daily life. Over the course of these pages, we'll discover that, although these practices emerged from one of the world's great spiritual traditions, the practical benefits of mantra and chanting are very much grounded in the real world.

How to Best Use This Book

The three parts of this book—Mindful Singing, Music and Mantras, and Songbook for the Soul—are intentionally arranged and sequenced to guide and support you on a progressively deepening journey of self-discovery.

In Part One: Mindful Singing, we'll learn about the amazing, life-enhancing benefits that singing has to offer each and every one of us, discovering how it can improve our physical, emotional, and psychological well-being. We'll uncover and explore our own innate musical gifts that we may not have even known we had. Most importantly, we'll discover a wealth of simple and effective vocal tools and practices through which we can easily find and express our own true voice—setting the stage for us to mindfully sing ourselves more fully into health, happiness, peace, and prosperity.

In Part Two: Music and Mantras, we'll take our newfound connection with our voice and begin to explore the powerful transformational energies and archetypes of mantra chanting. We'll discover how the latest insights of neuroscience can enliven and empower this ancient yogic practice in new and inspiring ways. We'll be introduced to the three modes of mantra practice and learn the unique qualities and benefits of each, revealing a variety of accessible ways in which to experience this healing and life-changing practice for ourselves. We'll begin this section with my own journey through music and mantra, an adventure that took me all the way from the smoky stage of a jazz club to the pristine, peaceful environment of a mountain ashram.

Part Three: Songbook for the Soul offers us an abundance of mantra and chanting practices of all kinds to explore, complete with links to audio recordings for us to follow along with and learn. We'll get acquainted with the sacred, vibrational language of Sanskrit—the "language of the Gods"—perhaps finding that we have much more in common with this ancient language than we realized. We'll dive into the radiant archetypes of the Deities—Ganesh, Lakshmi, Hanuman, Shakti, and Shiva—discovering how the inner meanings of their symbolism and the universal energies of love, peace, and wisdom that they embody can become our energetic allies in our own journey of healing and awakening.

Although the sections of this book are intended to be experienced in order, you may find yourself inspired to jump right into a mantra practice even as you're still exploring Part One or Part Two. If so, feel free to skip ahead to Part Three: Songbook for the Soul to find a mantra practice that resonates with you. You can begin your new mantra practice and then simply return to where you left off earlier in the book, continuing your way through the chapters.

Also, if you happen to come across any new and unfamiliar words as your journey through *Music and Mantras* unfolds, you'll find the Glossary at the end of the book to be a helpful resource you can refer to anytime you'd like. Similarly, the Recommended Resources Guide is another valuable reference you can turn to for further information on a wide variety of mantra- and chanting-related resources. And while you're in the neighborhood, you can also learn all about the history of one the most popular musical instruments in the mantra and chanting community—the harmonium—in the appendix entitled "A Note on the Harmonium."

Now, please join me on a journey of discovery to experience the joy of mindful singing, music, and mantras.

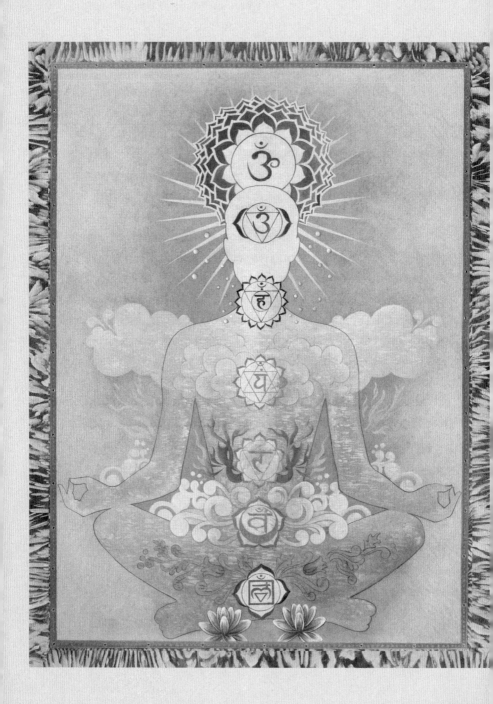

PART ONE

Mindful Singing

Chapter 1

Discovering My Voice

Singing is the rawest thing. Having been naked in films or naked in photo shoots, it's nothing compared to singing. It's absolute nakedness. You are stripped bare! It's very strange. Acting seems much easier, in fact, because you are putting on a costume—whereas here, you are taking everything off.

—Lou Doillon

I can speak from experience that our singing voice is deeply entwined with our core identities, a kind of shamanic tool that we can use to explore and heal the hidden parts of ourselves. Before I released my first album, *Reveal*, in 2004, I had never really shared my singing voice publicly. Singing for me had been a lifelong dream that, up to that point, had only found expression in the devotional chanting practices that were an essential part of my daily spiritual life. Chanting with the harmonium (Indian reed organ) in front of my home altar was and still is a deeply personal, intimate expression of singing. In that setting, it's just you and Spirit; you can sing freely, just for the joy of it. However, singing like that in front of a room full of people was something altogether new and unfamiliar.

I knew I had a profound calling to sing and to share these songs that were coming forth like musical flowers from this living plant of daily chanting practice that I'd been nurturing for more than a decade. Just after returning to California after my second trip to India, at a time when I was making part of my living as a professional *tabla* (Indian hand drums) player and had just recorded *Live on Earth* with Krishna Das, I awoke to the sound of that calling loud and clear in the form of an inner voice that said, *Unless you sing, you'll never truly be happy*. My mind did a quick fast-forward through a hypothetical version of my life that didn't include singing, and I saw with utter clarity that, at the end, I would be filled with regret that I hadn't taken this leap of faith to free my voice.

That day, I put aside the tablas I'd been practicing devotedly for three to four hours daily, resolved that I could still keep my drumming skills intact with just an hour a day or so. In their place, I began the journey of finding my voice—spending hours every day singing with my harmonium or guitar, practicing the Indian *sargam* vocal scales I had learned at the Ali Akbar College of Music, writing new mantra-based songs (beginning with the song *Ma*), and even taking a few voice lessons here and there to help guide me on my way. Most of all, I dove deeper and deeper into my daily chanting practice. That practice formed the foundation for the way I approached singing and fueled the inspiration for the songs that came through me.

When *Reveal* was released in 2004, the fifty-four minutes of music on that first album were the songs born from that period in my life. Even though I'd already been through the process of writing, recording, and producing at that point, until *Reveal* hit the streets, those songs and, more importantly, my singing voice, had so far existed solely in a kind of protective bubble into which only

I, my family, and the musicians and singers who recorded with me had been allowed. As far as everyone else was concerned, I was still the little drummer boy who played tablas for *kirtan* (a form of call-and-response chanting) singers like Krishna Das or Wah. It was one thing to sing at home or even in the recording studio but, with the release of *Reveal*, it felt as if I was allowing my voice to be heard by anyone in the world who chose to listen. On one hand, I felt exuberant to finally be able to share this musical offering and to let the world know that the little drummer boy had found his voice. On the other hand, putting this music out for everyone to hear felt a bit like walking down Santa Monica Boulevard stark naked in broad daylight. You can see why the album title was an obvious choice.

The very same week that *Reveal* came out, I had another debut of sorts, this one in the form of a red rash that appeared suddenly all over my neck, chest, and back. A friend who saw me around that time took a look at my red, inflamed neck and said, "Oh, wow. You look like you could be a Cardassian from *Star Trek*. It's kind of cool, actually." Finding myself inexplicably covered in a red, itchy rash was definitely not cool, however, because just as this new phase of my musical life was getting under way, the discomfort of this bizarre skin issue had suddenly made my day-to-day reality a challenge. I found it hard to sleep at night and even the touch of a shirt against my chest was incredibly irritating. I was miserable.

After a couple of visits to Western doctors, it became clear that the only strategy they were really offering was to suppress the rash temporarily with steroids—not a long-term solution. So, I set about looking for a more holistic approach that held out the possibility of real healing. I found a great acupuncturist/ herbalist in Los Angeles and went in for the initial consultation.

She examined me and listened sympathetically as I rattled off my litany of symptoms for her. At the end of that very first session, she reassured me and said she was confident that we could resolve whatever was creating this imbalance in my body through herbs, acupuncture, and dietary changes. I felt the first glimmer of hope that I might finally get some relief from the suffering I'd been going through. That's when she dropped a bit of holistic jujitsu on me: "You know, in Chinese medicine, we like to say that an illness is the body's way of asking you a question. Maybe your question is, 'Are you comfortable in your own skin?'"

Those words landed like a big stone in the middle of a lake, sending ripples out in every direction. It suddenly dawned on me that what was going on with my skin could be a kind of dramatic externalization of an underlying psychological or energetic blockage that was just coming to the surface—literally—to be healed. I felt daunted at the prospect that my healing from this uncomfortable condition wouldn't come in the form of a quick-fix prescription but, instead, would require me to evolve somehow, to embody myself more fully. Even so, I felt a sense of confidence and strength begin to come over me because I knew that I had a powerful ally to help me through the process: my singing and chanting practice.

Over the next nine months, with *Reveal* starting to find its way into the iPods and ears of people all around California and then beyond, I began playing my first concerts as a singer, still contending with the discomfort of the rash. At first, singing in front of an audience felt strange and a little intimidating, but the more I tried to cultivate the same feeling I would have chanting alone in front of my altar, the more natural and comfortable it felt. I began to notice that, while I was deeply in that sacred space of chanting, all the discomfort from the rash would vanish. At the end of those nine months, during a kirtan on the Big Island of Hawaii, the redness and irritation that had been my constant companion and fierce teacher for the better part of a year finally disappeared from my body.

Finding Your Voice

At this point I feel like I should insert one of those caveats you see at the end of those stock market trading services commercials with the message, "These results are not typical. Actual results will vary." Just to put your mind at ease, among the thousands of people I've encountered who've taken the journey to find their true voice, so far I'm the only one whose process included a temporary Cardassian neck tattoo. What finding our voice does give each and every one of us, though, is an opportunity to know ourselves more fully. Through the physical aspect of learning how to sing, we become more deeply aware of this physical instrument of our body; we begin to tune in to the deeper patterns of thought and feeling within us, and how those patterns are showing up in our body. By tuning into ourselves in this way through singing, we have a place from which we start expressing and releasing things. It's simple and direct.

The powerful transformative effect of releasing our voice is familiar territory for music therapists like Daniel Comstock, the director for the Center for Attitudinal Healing & the Arts in Montana. He describes the process of singing in a safe, judgment-free environment as an opportunity for our mind, body, and emotions to join, to come into alignment, which allows for healing. "If I'm aware that I'm using my body to express my emotions, then it's easier to let those emotions out. Well, if I'm singing a good piece of music or singing a chant that resonates with me, then those feelings start flowing through me. They stop being blocked. They stop being held. A good song along with a good sense of being fully in your body will start that process because you're connecting with yourself. By connecting with yourself, the truth of you—which is love—is going to be experienced and manifested. For me, my relationship to God and to the Universe is found through these actual concrete experiences of breathing and healing and singing and being and loving."[1]

As we embark on this healing journey to connect with our own singing voice, we'll begin with some amazing and inspiring insights about the power of singing. We'll discover how it's possible for the heartbeats of a group of singers to actually sync up to the same cardiovascular rhythm. We'll learn whether or not amateur singers can reap the same or even greater benefits from singing than professionals. And we'll see what an ancient Buddhist mantra has in common with the Christian *Ave Maria* prayer. In the next chapter, we'll explore together exactly how singing, chanting, and mantra affect our physical, emotional, and psychological well-being, our adaptability and longevity, and how we can cultivate and boost those life-enhancing properties of these fun and functional practices.

· ·

Music expresses that which cannot be put into words and that which cannot remain silent.
—VICTOR HUGO

· ·

Chapter 2

The Science of Singing

Healing is communication; and music, in its universal nature, is total communication. In the deepest mysteries of music are the inspirations, the pathways, and the healing which lead to oneness and unity.

—Olivea Dewhurst-Maddock

One of the most powerful qualities of mantra and chanting practice is that it opens the door into singing and musical experience for everyone, regardless of whether or not we bring any musical training or background to the table. This fact alone demonstrates chanting's immense value as a powerful tool to cultivate well-being and happiness. I like to think of chanting as a means of attuning our individual Self to the universal energy of life, like a violinist adjusting her instrument to be in tune with the orchestra. To carry that metaphor further, we could see the challenges in our lives as a kind of musical dissonance, a note that's a little (or a lot) off pitch and just needs some tuning up in the instrument of our physical, mental, emotional, or energetic bodies.

If we listen for it, we can hear this musical sensibility in common, everyday phrases. We say of a wise friend, "She's really tuned in." When we're feeling down we might say, "I've got the blues." If we're getting along well with someone, we might say, "We have a harmonious relationship." If someone insists on doing things his way, we might say, "He marches to the beat of a different drummer." And how could Austin Powers appropriately express his enthusiastic approval without his ever-present catchphrase, "Groovy, baby!"

Beyond these common expressions, it's easy to see that music is woven into the very fabric of our lives and memories. You only have to recall that favorite tune you loved as a child, or the love song that became the soundtrack for your first high school romance, or the music you chose to celebrate your first dance at your wedding. We each have a list of songs that pack a lot of joyful, happy memories, as well as songs that mark a sad or heart-breaking moment. Songs have the power to express what we feel inside, giving words and tone to our experience when we might find it difficult to communicate otherwise. We sing to mark occasions and celebrations, like birthdays and holidays. We sing in the shower, in our cars, to serenade our beloved; and parents all over the world know the power of singing to their babies—lullabies that soothe and comfort.

These musical expressions and experiences are a testament to the fact that music permeates life, not just as the soundtrack playing in the background but as an integral part of the human experience that's literally woven into our very biology. Each and every one of us, whether we know it yet or not, is a deeply musical being. My hope is that, even if we haven't discovered the musical side of ourselves yet, by the time we've finished this chapter we'll be fully convinced that it's there and that we can benefit tremendously by nurturing it.

Tuning Up

Let's take a moment to appreciate just how tuned in to music and sound the human organism really is. First, consider the sense of hearing itself, which is one of the first to develop in utero and the last to leave at the time of death. Now, consider the fact that these amazing ears of ours come standard with an intricately tuned pitch-recognition network within them called a tonotopic map (from the Greek, meaning "the place of tones") that enables us to process and recognize specific sound frequencies, sending them on to different parts of the brain depending on their particular pitch. Then, to process that information, specific cells in the brain consistently light up in response to one particular frequency or a multiple of that frequency. Incredibly, human beings can process these tones with absolutely no musical training whatsoever! What's more, for about one out of ten thousand people this ability is so pronounced that they can correctly identify the name of any frequency they hear. Someone with this gift of "perfect frequency" can hear a tone and, without any conscious thought, recognize it as middle C, for example, just like you and I might look at the grass and recognize that it's green.

It's inspiring to realize that this inborn musicality exists in all of us, whether or not we're born with perfect pitch, as the neuroscientist Dr. Daniel Levitin discovered back in 1990. He took forty non-musicians and recorded them singing their favorite songs from memory. What he discovered was astounding. The majority of his subjects sang the songs at or close to the actual pitch of the original recorded version. Then, when he asked them to sing a second song, they did it again. Remember, these were all non-musicians.

The icing on the cake, though, was Dr. Levitin's observation that these subjects not only replicated the correct pitch of the original recordings but were often able to replicate many of the little vocal nuances from their chosen songs as well (Michael Jackson's falsetto "ee-hee" from his song "Billie Jean," for instance). In his book *This Is Your Brain on Music*, he describes just how musical these "non-musicians" really were: "I created a tape that had the subjects' productions on one channel of a stereo signal and the original recording on the other. It sounded as though the subjects were singing along with the record, but we hadn't played the record to them, they were singing along with the memory representation in their head, and that memory representation was astonishingly accurate."[2]

As we can see, the truth is that all human beings are musical. Yes, some have taken the time to cultivate the specific skills required to master a musical instrument while others haven't. Regardless of that, however, with or without the cultivation of those very specific skills, we are all—each and every one of us—musical beings.

In my travels around the world I've witnessed countless times how virtually everyone—including folks who've never touched a musical instrument or ventured to sing outside of their car or their shower—can discern whether a string on a guitar is in tune or out of tune with the other strings. (Thank you, tonotopic map!) When we walk down the aisles of the grocery store feeling inexplicably stoked as we bop along to the sounds of *Upbeat Hits of the 90s* pumping through the speakers above our heads, it's because our brains are having an automatic, unconscious, and very musical response by becoming entrained by the rhythms of the music. Whether or not we're big fans of C+C Music Factory, once that groove starts we're nodding our heads, tapping our toes, maybe even singing along while we try to find a ripe avocado because our brains are feeling the groove, too, sending out neurochemical messages to our entire body that say, *Everybody dance now!*

As we progress further into this chapter, we'll see how our human biology is also particularly responsive and attuned to singing, especially in a group. Scientists are still trying to understand exactly why this is the case but some have theorized that it's an evolutionary adaptation based on singing's role in social bonding. Way back when humans began to shift from the nomadic, solitary culture of our ancient past in favor of gathering together in larger, collective groups, there had to be a way to bond the various members of that group together so that there was cooperation and harmony rather than every caveman for himself.

According to Dr. Eiluned Pearce, an evolutionary neuroscientist from the University of Oxford, that social bonding was traditionally a one-on-one interaction (like when we see the members of a troop of monkeys patiently grooming one another), but when human societies began to form, the larger population made one-to-one bonding inefficient and difficult. However, Pearce says, "you could imagine some kind of singing ritual to bond groups together very quickly so they could then take part in some sort of collective activity like hunting. Group singing involves a shared group goal and synchronous activity. It has also previously been shown to trigger the release of chemicals in the brain that might facilitate bonding."[3]

When we sing, especially when we sing with a group, our brain releases some very particular hormones that unleash a cascade of warm, fuzzy feelings in us. Those hormones include the endorphin dopamine, a neurotransmitter with psychoactive properties that floods us with pleasurable sensations—nature's way of rewarding us for behaviors such as making love and eating that are integral to our survival (aka, the "biological imperative"). Singing also triggers the release of the neurotransmitter oxytocin—the very same hormone produced by the brains of women during childbirth and breastfeeding, as well as by the brains of both men and women at the moment of orgasm—which alleviates anxiety and stress while inspiring feelings of trust and bonding.

We can see already that singing and music are intricately woven into the fabric of our biology and our lives. Now let's explore some of the other well-known, scientifically measurable effects and benefits of music and singing.

The Science of Singing

Research in neuroscience, psychology and medicine as well as in music education, cultural studies, social sciences and the history of emotion shows the immense impact of singing on human development. Not only does singing have positive effects on synapse formations in the brain and on bodily functions and emotional well-being, it also creates strong, felt communities that have the power to shape both individuals and societies.

—DR. MARIE LOUISE HERZFELD-
SCHILD AND PHILIPPE RIXHON

In 2005, the University of Sheffield, UK, conducted a study of the effects of singing in groups. Although some of the participants in the study did have some musical background, one of the main points of focus for the research was to try to measure the effects of singing on non-musicians. To this end, the researchers actually assembled a choir of homeless people with no musical training whatsoever. The results of their study couldn't have been clearer: "Group singing and performance, even at the most amateur levels of musicality, yielded considerable emotional, social and cognitive benefits."[4]

One of the greatest gifts of singing in the context of a chanting practice is that it provides us a judgment-free zone in which to open our voices. We can sing simply for the joy of it as an expression of our love, our gratitude, our highest aspirations and intentions, with absolutely no thought of whether we're "good" singers or what someone else might think of our voice. As this study shows, the considerable benefits that come from singing are not tied to any arbitrary measurement of musical quality.

Stop for a moment and truly appreciate the astronomical odds that had to play out in precisely the right way, at precisely the right time, and in precisely the right place for life to bring forth this human being called *you*, just as you are this very minute. When we open our mouths and sing, we can choose to really feel just how miraculous we truly are. We can sing with the awareness that—no matter what any other person happens to think about our voice, no matter even what *we* might happen to think about our voice—as far as the Universe is concerned, our voice is music to its ears. And, if you like, you can replace the word *Universe* with *Spirit, God, Divine Mother*, or whatever feels right.

··

> There is no "good" singing, there
> is only present and absent.
> —JEFF BUCKLEY

··

The Heart of the Matter

A group of researchers in Sweden conducted a series of scientific studies in 2013 documenting the powerfully beneficial effect that singing has on human health and resiliency. The study focused on singing's dramatic effects on one of the most telling indicators of overall well-being and adaptability in humans, something called heart rate variability, or HRV. According to the HeartMath Institute, "Numerous studies show HRV is a key indicator of physiological resiliency and behavioral flexibility, and can reflect an ability to adapt effectively to stress and environmental demands."[5]

In this Swedish study, a group of fifteen young singers came into the lab and researchers measured the biological changes that occurred when they hummed, sang hymns, and chanted mantras as a group. The scientists found that, although all three forms of singing definitely produced improvements in the singers' HRV, the most significant benefits were measured when the participants were chanting mantras. And that's not all. The researchers also found that these changes in the singers' hearts were happening in the same way at the same time among the members of the group. The heart rates of the group were syncing up with one another!

Björn Vickhoff, the leader of the study, concludes: "Singing regulates activity in the vagus nerve, which is involved in our emotional life and our communication with others. Songs with long phrases achieve the same effect as breathing exercises in yoga. It's a beautiful thing to feel. You are not alone but with others who feel the same way."[6]

If you've had the amazing experience of attending a kirtan, a call-and-response form of mantra practice, where you've felt as if the energy of everyone in the room had come together into an ecstatic wave of joy, the findings of this and other studies point to an internal counterpart to that felt, external experience. It just may be that when we sing and chant together in a group like this our hearts really do beat as one.

· ·

When you sing with a group of people . . . it's all about the immersion of the self into the community. That's one of the great feelings—to stop being "me" for a while and to become "us." That way lies empathy—the great social virtue.

—BRIAN ENO

· ·

Jesus and Buddha on the Mainline

Shedding even more light on the powerful effects of singing and chanting, a research study conducted in Italy in 2001 zeroed in on two mantras from completely different spiritual traditions: the *Ave Maria* rosary prayer and the Buddhist mantra *Om Mani Padme Hum*. Twenty-three subjects chanted together as a group while the researchers measured their bodies' responses using state-of-the-art technology. Once again, the beneficial heart rate variability measurement improved as the group sang either chant and, once again, the group's heart rate oscillations synced up together.

However, the Italian study went a step further in trying to pinpoint exactly why this particular form of chanting has such a potent effect in enhancing this key indicator of human health, well-being, and adaptability. In measuring the respiration rates of the subjects as they chanted, the researchers discovered that—despite the fact that these two chants come from traditions that are worlds apart—they each produce an almost identical breathing pattern in the chanters. Whether they were chanting *Ave Maria* or *Om Mani Padme Hum*, the subjects' breathing was slowed down to around six breaths per minute, whereas normal breathing is usually around fifteen breaths per minute. The researchers believe that this slower respiration rate of six breaths per minute is synchronizing the chanters' breath with a powerful, naturally occurring circulatory rhythm known as the Mayer wave (essentially, a ten-second cycle in blood pressure). Aligning our breathing with this internal circulatory pulse has been shown to produce feelings of calm and well-being, while enhancing and improving both respiratory and cardiovascular function. According to the researchers, this alignment between the breath and the heart that singing these chants produced was no accident. "We believe that the rosary may have partly evolved because it synchronized with the inherent cardiovascular (Mayer) rhythms, and thus gave a feeling of well-being, and perhaps an increased responsiveness to the religious message."

They also point to the fact that the particular style of chanting of the *Ave Maria* rosary is not typical of other Christian prayers, and that there's some historical evidence to support the idea that this style of chanting actually originated with Tibetan monks and Indian yogis. According to the authors of the study, the rosary came to Europe with the crusaders, by way of the Middle East, by way of Tibet and India. Regardless of the rosary's original heritage, both chants certainly evolved in an era before the invention of mechanical timekeeping devices, so "a rhythmic formula was the easiest way to keep a reasonably accurate timing in the range of several seconds per breath, and thus a good way to learn to slow respiration to a given rate. The benefits of respiratory exercises to slow respiration in the practice of yoga have long been reported, and mantras may have evolved as a simple device to slow respiration, improve concentration and induce calm."[7]

We can all experience the beneficial effects of this form of chanting for ourselves with any mantra singing practice that aligns us with that magical rhythm of six breaths per minute. Any chant we sing that has about a ten-second phrase per breath will get us in the zone. And while this particular study measured the effects of this style of chanting on a group of singers, we'll still receive all the same benefits even if we're chanting completely solo on our own.

You can experience this incredibly powerful form of singing for yourself when you reach the end of the chapter called "The Yoga of Mindful Singing" at the end of Part One of the book. There, you'll be introduced to the 5-Minute *Om* practice, complete with an audio link you can sing along with. In addition, you'll find a special version of the *Om Namah Shivaya* mantra in the Songbook for the Soul section at the end of the book. By singing along with the audio link, you'll learn the beautiful, slow style of chanting this mantra that flows perfectly with this powerful breathing rhythm.

While the 5-Minute *Om* practice and the slow *Om Namah Shivaya* mantra are great introductions to this particular form of chanting practice, there are others as well. Many of the text chants we'll learn in the Songbook for the Soul can also work well with this style of chanting, provided we adjust our breathing accordingly. The *Hanuman Chalisa*, *Devi Suktam*, and *Nirvanashatkam*, for example, all fit perfectly into this slower breathing rhythm, provided we take our inhalation every other line.

....

When you're singing, you're using extra muscles, and it requires a lot of exercise and breathing. You can't do that if you're a sissy. If I have any fitness advice for people, I'd tell them to sing more. It's good therapy, too.

—WILLIE NELSON

....

Sing, Sing a Song

Mindful of the undeniable benefits that singing can bring to our physical, mental, and emotional health, the National Endowment for the Arts partnered with George Washington University and other national arts organizations in 2006 to demonstrate how those benefits might serve older, retirement-age adults. Over the course of two years, there were three hundred subjects, age sixty-five and older, who participated in a "Creativity and Aging Study" in sites located in Washington, Brooklyn, and San Francisco. After a thorough intake exam and assessment to match up their overall level of health and functioning, the group was divided in half: 150 of the subjects would become the control group and would just go on with life as they had been, while the other 150 subjects began participating in weekly arts programs that included choir singing, music, dance, poetry, and more.

To get a sense of just how spectacularly successful the music and arts programs were at boosting the health and well-being of these participants as compared to the control group, consider the stated expectations set out by the researchers at the start of the study. Given that the average age of the participants was eighty years old, "clinicians and researchers alike would generally consider interventions in this age group successful, in terms of positive health and social functioning effects, if there was *less decline* than expected over time in the intervention group as compared to control group."[8] In other words, the consensus bar for defining success was set down low at, "Okay, they're declining *less* quickly than expected. Hooray!"

But these geriatric rock stars shattered the researchers' expectations. Just one year into the two-year study—far from merely declining less—the subjects in the arts and music group were already reporting *improvements* in their health, well-being, and functioning. Those improvements just kept right on gathering steam over the course of the second year as well. When it was all said and done and the results were compiled, the groovy grandparents in the music and art group had left the control group in the dust. Here's a partial list of the results of the study:

- **Overall Health:** The art group reported a noticeable improvement in their overall health and well-being, while the control group reported a decline.
- **Doctor's Visits:** The art group reported a significant decrease in the number of doctor's visits, while the control group reported an increase.
- **Medications:** The art group reported using less prescription as well as over-the-counter medications, while the control group reported using more.
- **Depression:** The art group got better marks on the depression assessment, while those in the control group did less well.
- **Social Participation:** The art group reported an increase in the amount of social activities they were engaged in, while the control group stayed the same or declined.

The incredible results of this study seem to have even amazed the scientists who conducted it. In their conclusion, the researchers describe the remarkable changes they observed in their subjects through the "powerful positive intervention effects" of the music and arts programs. In italics, the scientists dramatically emphasize that the study demonstrates the "true health promotion and disease prevention effects" of music and arts, and assert that for older adults these activities "appear to be reducing risk factors that drive the need for long-term care."[9]

> When we are weighed down by deep despondency, we should for a while sing psalms out loud, raising our voice with joyful expectation until the thick mist is dissolved by the warmth of song.
>
> —ST. DIADOCHOS OF PHOTIKI

Inspired by the findings of the "Creativity and Aging Study," the National Institutes of Health (NIH) is funding further research at UC San Francisco, zeroing in solely on the therapeutic effects of group singing in a five-year study that's under way right now in 2016. The researchers are exploring the very real possibility that singing in a community choir program could be an economical way to cultivate greater health and well-being in older adults. The director of the research, a cognitive neuroscientist named Dr. Julene Johnson, says the goal of the study is "to provide scientific-based evidence" that community-based group singing can promote greater physical, emotional, and social health. This current study is a continuation of earlier research she conducted as a Fulbright Scholar in Finland, where she and her team documented a strong correlation between choir singing and quality of life for older adults.[10]

Now, let's just take a step back and consider for a moment that the NIH—America's primary agency in charge of all health-related research and one of the world's preeminent medical research centers, period—has seen fit to invest its research dollars into a serious scientific study focused on singing. In the face of soaring health care costs and a population that is living longer than ever before in human history, the goal of an agency like the NIH is to research and discover novel and cost-effective ways to support health and well-being. Like their website says, the NIH exists to "turn discoveries into health." Well, at this very moment this prestigious organization is betting their research dollars on group singing, confident that the benefits they find will lead to discoveries they can turn into health practices for everyone.

While the San Francisco study is focused on gathering scientific proof of the benefits that singing can offer to senior citizens, those benefits are by no means limited to any particular age group. In *Time* magazine's article entitled "Singing Changes Your Brain" they shared the stunning statistics on just how popular group singing has become for folks across all generations. According to the article, in 2013, more than 32 million Americans were singing gleefully in some 270,000 different community chorus groups around the country. That's an increase of about 10 million singers since the last survey taken six years prior. The choruses that *Time* mentioned ran the stylistic gamut from gospel hymns to show tunes to vocal arrangements of pop music favorites.[11]

If they had asked me, I would have gladly drawn their attention to the blossoming renaissance of another one of the world's most tried-and-true forms of group singing whose participants could have dramatically increased the ranks of their choir count as well, a tradition of call-and-response chanting that began more than 1,300 years ago in medieval India. I'm talking, of course, about kirtan.

In addition to the multitude of proven benefits we've already learned that any form of group singing already has to offer, kirtan goes one better by enhancing the experience with a few powerful and unique ingredients. First, kirtan is often sung in Sanskrit, one of the world's sacred languages. While it's true that your average kirtan attendee may or may not understand a word of Sanskrit, the energetic and vibrational qualities of this ancient, sacred language truly speak for themselves. Secondly, the simple call-and-response style of kirtan allows everyone—even complete beginners—to feel at home with this very accessible practice. Finally, kirtan leaves aside the typical lyrical content of other forms of singing in favor of repeating the "Names of God." The positive energies and archetypes these Names express and embody inspire uplifting thoughts and feelings in the chanters. Taken all together, these unique qualities of kirtan combine to create a powerfully joyful and ecstatic singing experience. Like the blossoming choir movement, kirtan's natural appeal has attracted many enthusiastic participants and this chanting practice that originated in seventh-century India is now enjoyed in yoga and spiritual communities all over America and around the world.

With the myriad benefits to physical health, emotional and psychological well-being, and overall human happiness that singing and chanting have to offer, it's easy to see why we would want to invite more and more of this amazing and accessible practice into our lives. To fully experience the wide variety of mantras and chants that we'll learn together in this book, we'll want to begin by connecting with and strengthening our own unique singing voice. In the chapters that follow, we'll take this essential first step—awakening and expressing our true voice—as we continue our unfolding journey of self-discovery through mindful singing.

Chapter 3

The Drone Zone

Since the one thing we can say about fundamental
matter is that it is vibrating, and since all vibrations
are theoretically sound, then it is not unreasonable
to suggest that the universe is music and should be
perceived as such.

—Joachim-Ernst Berendt

In this chapter we'll get acquainted with a powerful ally for
our singing, chanting, and meditation practice—the musical
drone. In the world of music, a drone is simply one or more
notes that sustain over the entire course of a musical piece, giving a resonant harmonic foundation upon which the music can
unfold. For us, as mindful singers and chanters, the incredible
support that a drone provides spans several different areas. First,
a musical drone supports our intonation in singing by providing a crystal-clear reference to pitch. Second, the drone acts as
a kind of "third lung" that seems to bolster and strengthen our
own voice by vibrating in harmony with it. And finally, even
when our mantra practice is silent and internal, as when we're
doing *japa* (internal mantra repetition), the drone can help to

settle and focus the mind through its calming and harmonizing vibrations.

One of the signature sounds of Indian classical music is produced by the *tamboura*, a beautiful stringed instrument that resembles a large lute. Although most tambouras are quite ornate and elegant, the bulb-like base of the instrument is traditionally made from a simple, hollowed-out pumpkin gourd. In a centuries-old musical tradition that boasts the likes of Ravi Shankar, Ali Akbar Khan, Zakir Hussain, and other virtuosos, it may be surprising to learn that one of the essential instruments of that tradition never plays anything other than the two notes to which it's usually tuned. While the maestro on *sitar* or *sarod*, two other Indian classical music instruments, burns up the stage with his or her musical fireworks, the tamboura simply drones its two notes quietly, steadily, in the background.

Let's experience the tamboura drone for ourselves by following the audio link:

Tamboura Drone in C: GirishMusic.com/BookAudio

As you listen to the sound of the tamboura drone, pay special attention to the resonant, scintillating quality of the instrument. You may notice that the sound of the drone seems to flow in undulating waves of vibration, which is part of the enchanting quality of the tamboura that makes it such an effective support for chanting and meditation practice. You might also imagine the low, resonating sound of the tamboura playing in the background of Indian classical music like that of Ravi Shankar, creating a sonic canvas to feature the melodic pluck of the sitar. You'd be right to think that one of the most advanced musical systems in the world didn't elevate the simple tamboura to such a central role by accident. And understanding how the tamboura came to hold such a prominent position in Indian music might just inspire us to embrace this musical ally as well in our own journey with mindful singing and mantra.

One of the unique qualities of Indian music that sets it apart from most Western pop, jazz, or classical is that, rather than moving through a series of different chords (sing "Happy Birthday to You," for a good example), the majority of Indian music instead zeroes in on one single scale, or *raga*, exploring the various nuances and harmonic relationships that are possible within it.

The overall quality of this style of music, called "dronal" music, might best be described as introspective and even trance-inducing. Without the distraction of changing chords, the mind can more easily sink into deep states of absorption through listening to the subtly blossoming permutations of the raga, all while held in the steady sonic firmament of the tamboura drone. Whereas the typically chord-based music of the West could be described as "horizontal"—moving from here to there to there and back again—one might say that Indian dronal music is more "vertical"—exploring the heights and depths of a singular yet intricate tapestry of sound.

The intoxicating sonic allure of the tamboura moved me to such heights that, on my second trip to India, I shelled out around 18,000 rupees (about $300) and purchased one from the Rikhi Ram music store in New Delhi. And even though the prices in India are famously low, shlepping a large, stringed instrument around in taxis, trains, and planes to get it back home to California turned out to be a rather grueling ordeal. Although the tamboura and I did indeed make it home intact, I'm thrilled to report that there are far simpler ways to get your drone on—ones that don't require passports, visas, or bearing the uncomfortable stares of customs agents.

Digital Drones

Welcome to the world of the digital drone! In the era of the Internet, iTunes, and apps, the tamboura drone—in any key you'd like—is literally right at your fingertips. (Did I mention that a real tamboura is large, fragile, and requires constant, careful tuning?) With a little searching, you'll be up to your ears in the exquisite sounds of the tamboura—one of the greatest allies you'll find for supporting and inspiring your chanting or meditation practice. Please note that, like a lot of other words translated from Sanskrit, *tamboura* is sometimes spelled differently. *Tanpura* and *tambura* are also common variations referring to exactly the same instrument, so keep that in mind as you peruse the worldwide dronescape.

Let's look at a few of the tamboura drone resources that I've discovered over the years so that you can begin exploring on your own. A quick note: whereas the recordings mentioned below feature tambouras tuned to only one or, at most, two keys, a tamboura app will allow you to easily set your tuning to any key you'd like with the push of a button. So, if you imagine that you'd like to have the freedom to "dial a drone" in the key of your choice, you'll want to go with one of the apps. We'll discuss how to go about choosing the best key for you a little later in the chapter.

Below is a list of a few of my favorite tamboura drone resources for you to explore.

Tamboura CDs and MP3s

Tamboura: Music for Deep Meditation, from Inner Splendor Media and Banyan Education. An excellent-quality recording of a tamboura drone in the key of B-flat.

Deep Relaxation with the Celestial Sound of the Tamboura, also from Inner Splendor. This recording features three tracks— tamboura drone in D with a low synth drone, tamboura in B-flat with Tibetan bells, and a track of pure tamboura in D.

Tamboura Apps

iTanpura Pro: This is my go-to tamboura app at the moment. It features great-sounding tamboura samples and, because this app uses two tambouras playing simultaneously, the drone is very smooth and seamless. It's a bit pricier than some of the other apps but definitely worth it. You can try a free, limited-function version of the app called *iTanpura Lite* if you'd like to check it out before you buy. (The *Lite* version has all the functionality of the pro version except the drone will automatically stop after one minute of play.)

RealTanpura: This app prides itself on "high-fidelity audio of a real acoustic tamboura." Although it does seem to have a fairly full, rich sound, it relies on only one tamboura and the drone isn't quite as smooth as iTanpura's.

iTabla Pandit: I recently discovered this all-in-one tamboura and tabla app, which I'm including in this list because of the uniquely deep and bassy tones of its drones. You'll want to try the free *Lite* version first because this bad boy is the priciest of the bunch in its full professional version. If you're a fan of lots of low end in your drone, you'll want to check this one out.

Tanpura Droid: This one's for Android device users and also goes for the two-tamboura approach, giving a nice, smooth drone in any key.

> There is geometry in the humming of the strings.
> There is music in the spacing of the spheres.
> —PYTHAGORAS

Getting Your Drone On

Once you're all set with your tamboura drone, whether you're using a recording or one of the apps listed above, there are a few things to be aware of so that you can fully experience the beauty of this ancient instrument. First, the sonic characteristics of the tamboura stretch across a very wide spectrum of the audio frequency range, from way down low in those warm, reverberating bass tones all the way up to those sparkly, crystalline highs on top. With that said, it's obvious that the dinky little speaker on an iPhone just isn't going to cut it for a sonic palette as wide-ranging as the tamboura's. You'll want to get your drone on in hi-fi, if possible, by plugging into a nice pair of stereo speakers or a reasonably good audio docking station. This is guaranteed to give you a more authentic, full-bodied experience of what this amazing instrument really sounds and feels like. When you sit next to an actual, live tamboura, you feel the vibrations tickling your spine and moving around the molecules in your body in a very good way indeed. As you're listening to your tamboura drone at home, set the volume to a moderate level so that it's not overwhelming but you can still feel the vibrations of the sound in your body.

Secondly, if you've ventured into the world of tamboura apps, you'll want to have a quick, simple tutorial in how to dial in the proper notes for the digital tamboura to play. Most of these apps have an abundance of features that can seem overwhelming at first. (*iTabla Pandit*, in particular, has a graphic display that looks like the control panel on a space shuttle or something.) Not to worry, though, because getting our basic drone up and running is as simple as pushing a couple of buttons. Let's give it a try:

1. **Select your key:** To begin with, you'll want to select what musical key or pitch you'll be droning in. This is as simple as pushing the main pitch buttons in the app up or down to get to the desired key. You'll see the pitch letter name (C, D, E, and so on) change in response. In the case of *iTabla Pandit*, you select your pitch by touching the actual name of the key directly, rather than using up or down buttons. For now, though, to keep things simple let's start in the key of C. All of the apps with the exception of *iTabla Pandit* automatically open in the key of C anyway, but now you know how to change your drone key if you'd like to. More about why you might want to do that in a moment.

2. **Select your drone interval:** Once you've chosen the key you'll be singing in, the next thing you'll want to do is to select the "harmonic interval" for your drone. Don't be alarmed, this is just a fancy way of saying "the other note

that your tamboura will play along with your main pitch."
Now, when it comes to tamboura drones, that other
note is typically the fifth note of the key you happen to
be playing in, otherwise known as the harmonic fifth.
Never heard of a harmonic fifth, you say? Well, I beg to
differ. If you would, kindly sing the first line of "Twinkle,
Twinkle, Little Star." Go ahead, I'll give you a moment.

Very good. The interval between the first and the second
"twinkle" that you just sang is what is known in musical parlance
as the harmonic fifth. The fifth holds a rather special place among
musical intervals because it is considered to be one of the most
harmonious and pleasing of all the intervals. The special qualities
of this musical interval have been noted by, among others, the
Greek mathematician and philosopher Pythagoras, who wrote
that the vibrations of the harmonic fifth had healing and restorative benefits. It's not surprising, then, that the harmonic fifth
is typically the interval of choice for tamboura drones in Indian
classical music, given this tradition's emphasis on spirituality and
introspection.

Now, getting back to our tamboura app, in order to find the
harmonic fifth, we'll need just one other bit of inside information
about Indian music. The names of the notes in the Indian scale system differ from the familiar *Do-Re-Mi* that Julie Andrews immor-
talized years ago in *The Sound of Music*. In the Indian version of
the musical scale, the first five notes are *Sa, Re, Ga, Ma*, and, most
importantly for our purposes here, *Pa*. These are the very same
notes as *Do, Re, Mi*, and so on but without the entertaining refer-
ences to female deer or hot beverages to enjoy with jam and bread.

Now that you're savvy to the Indian scale system, you can see
that selecting the harmonic fifth on our tamboura drone app is as

simple as tapping the *Pa* button. In the case of *iTanpura*, you'll tap it twice, once for each of the two tambouras.

To review, there are just two simple steps to get your digital drone on:

1. Use the pitch buttons to select your key (begin with C)
2. Tap the *Pa* buttons to choose the drone of the harmonic fifth.

Exploring Different Keys

Once you've gotten familiar with the basics of your drone app, you may feel inclined to venture out into other musical keys besides the familiar home base of C. There are a few factors that might inspire you to try some other drone keys, depending on what kind of practice you're doing and your own personal preferences.

First, if you're choosing a drone key to support your chanting and singing, you'll be best served to choose a drone key based on your own unique vocal instrument and where your voice feels most comfortable. I recommend going through the singing exercises in the chapter called "Finding Your Vocal Sweet Spot" to really tune in to your ideal key center. Essentially, though, you can simply tune in to how it feels to sing in a certain key. Does it feel like you're straining or tensing in your throat? If so, you might want to drop the pitch of the drone down. Or perhaps you notice that the drone feels a little too low and sleepy. In that case, you can simply raise the pitch a step or two at a time with the push of a button. Let your awareness be your guide and really tune in to how it feels to sing in a given key for you. You want to find your vocal home base so that singing there is always comfortable, relaxed, and open.

Secondly, if singing isn't on the menu and you're looking to choose a drone key to play in the background for your japa or other meditation practice, for instance, you're free to explore new territory of musical keys inspired by things other than your own vocal range. As one possible resource for inspiration, we can attune our drone key to a pitch that's aligned with a certain energetic quality or *chakra* (energy center). We might find that we can enhance our practice by aligning the energetic quality of the drone key in support of the issue or intention we're focused on in our practice. Here's a list of the musical tones associated with the seven chakras and the energies and qualities associated with them:

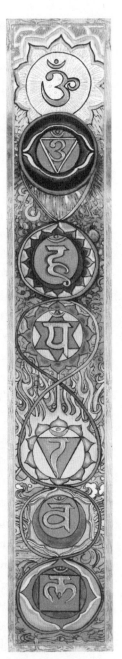

KEY	CHAKRA NAME	LOCATION	ELEMENT	ENERGY
C	1st Chakra (Muladhara)	Root	Earth	Grounding
D	2nd Chakra (Svadhisthana)	Sacrum	Water	Life-energy
E	3rd Chakra (Manipura)	Navel	Fire	Power
F	4th Chakra (Anahata)	Heart	Air	Love
G	5th Chakra (Vishuddha)	Throat	Ether	Creativity
A	6th Chakra (Ajna)	Third Eye	All	Wisdom/Insight
B	7th Chakra (Sahasrara)	Crown	All	Transcendence

You can use this list as a starting point for exploration to see what resonates for you in your practice. The pitch/element/energy correspondences above are simply a commonly used formula, they're not written in stone. So, again, let your own awareness be your guide in choosing the key that feels right for you. You may also find that the key that resonates for you this week is different than the one that felt right last week. Experiment and keep your ears and your mind open. In my own practice, I often choose to do my singing in the key of C, but I've found that I really resonate with the key of B for doing japa and meditation. Then again, I'm rather fond of the key of F. Since we have the luxury of simple push-button tuning with our digital drone rather than the cumbersome task of physically adjusting the wooden tuning pegs of an actual tamboura, the sky's the limit. Have fun!

The beautiful, healing sounds of the tamboura can be a powerful source of inspiration anytime we choose to invite it into our lives. Beyond its welcome, uplifting contribution to our chanting, mantra, or meditation in the sacred space of our home altar, yoga room, or wherever we've chosen to practice, we can also bring the inspiring vibrations of the tamboura out into our daily lives as well. Since the contemporary audio incarnation of this ancient musical instrument is so incredibly portable, there's no reason why we can't take our bliss on the road, literally.

As a substitute for the radio or other music in the car, why not immerse ourselves in the calming, centering sounds of the tamboura drone? We can *Om* or sing our favorite chants as we're out and about. It's an energizing and uplifting alternative that allows us to carry the energies of our chanting practice into our day-to-day routine. I've been known to sing the entire *Hanuman Chalisa* in my car while I'm out driving across the country on tour, with the sweet sounds of the tamboura drone carrying me along on my journey. Or perhaps we might find that a soft drone playing in the background in our living room at home can transform an ordinary environment into one that is infused with positive, healing vibrations.

In any way we might choose to invite the sounds of the tamboura drone into our lives, we are truly connecting with the ancient healing power of music and vibration.

As one listens to the resonance of the sounds of stringed instruments, he or she becomes absorbed in the space of eternal consciousness.

—FROM THE *VIJNANABHAIRAVA TANTRA*

Chapter 4

Finding Your Vocal Sweet Spot

The human voice is the organ of the soul.

—Henry Wadsworth Longfellow

In this chapter, we'll begin to explore our voices and discover our "vocal type." With this knowledge in hand, we'll tune in to our own, unique vocal sweet spot—our home base from which all of our singing and chanting practice can fully blossom.

This one-of-a-kind musical instrument that is your voice finds expression through your own equally unique body. Whether you're short or tall, male or female, narrow or wide—the size, shape, and structure of your body all come together to create a voice that is uniquely "you." Isn't it amazing that, out of all the millions of people in the world, a friend knows exactly who's calling just by hearing the sound of your voice on the telephone line?

Part of the journey we can take with singing and chanting practice is to better understand ourselves through the unique instrument of our own voice. Discovering our vocal type—which of the six general categories of the vocal range feels right for us—will be our first step on this journey.

Tuning to Your *Om* Base

Now, regardless of which vocal type we happen to be, each of us has an essential part to sing in the choir, metaphorically speaking. Even so, it's still really important to assign the right parts to the right singers! In other words, someone with the low vocal range of a bass simply won't be able to belt out those high soprano parts, and he just might hurt himself trying. So, let's begin by finding our actual place among these six zones within the landscape of the human voice.

Since this book is about opening our voices for chanting practice, healing, and our own personal enjoyment rather than, say, auditioning for a part on Broadway, we're not focused here on pushing the extremes of our vocal range. What we're really looking for is the place where our voice feels the most at home.

However, in the brief exercise below, we will spend just sixty seconds or so discovering the lowest low and the highest high that feels comfortable for us. Once we've identified the top and bottom ends of our unique vocal spectrum, we can more easily locate our middle ground, our sweet spot, our natural home base.

As you do the vocal type exercise below, pay special attention to your throat as you sing. Let it feel as relaxed and open as possible. Don't strain. Let's begin:

Vocal Type Exercise: GirishMusic.com/BookAudio

1. This exercise begins with a descending (progressively lower) series of notes. Sing "ah" along with each pitch until you reach the lowest note that you can sing

comfortably. Write this note down. This is your **Bottom Note**.

2. For the second part of the exercise, you'll hear an ascending (progressively higher) series of notes. Sing "ah" along with each pitch until you reach the highest note that you can sing comfortably. Write this note down. This is your **Top Note**.

3. If you weren't quite sure, replay the exercise and try it again a time or two until you're fairly confident in your answers.

4. Now, compare the top and bottom notes that you wrote down with the chart below. Keep in mind that men's voices typically fall into one of the first three categories (bass, baritone, or tenor) while women's voices usually fall into one of the last three (alto, mezzo soprano, or soprano).

VOCAL TYPE CHART

	BASS	BARITONE	TENOR	ALTO	MEZZO SOPRANO	SOPRANO
Top Note	C4	E4	G4	D5	F5	A5
Bottom Note	E2	G2	B2	F3	A3	C4

Ta-da! Congratulations, now you know your vocal type. It's okay if your top or low note was off by one from the chart, you'll still get a pretty clear indication of which vocal type you are. Now let's take this discovery and apply it to our singing and chanting practice.

Sweet Spot Vocal Types

As I mentioned before, the real purpose of the vocal type exercise is to find our home base as singers. Now that we know where we fit into the choir, let's zero in on that sweet spot—that middle ground where each of our unique voices can really blossom and express itself without strain or tension. Once we've discovered our vocal sweet spot, this will become our go-to musical key for whatever singing or chanting practices we'd like to do. If you don't happen to have your own harmonium or keyboard, you'll want to set yourself up with a digital tamboura drone app and follow the detailed instructions in the "Drone Zone" chapter for selecting your musical key of choice.

Using a tamboura drone, harmonium, or keyboard of any kind you like, refer to the suggested notes below as a starting point. You can move up or down by half steps from the suggested note—meaning the very next note on your keyboard, for example, or one tap of the up or down arrow buttons in your tamboura app—and explore singing long "ah"s.

Please note that in the Vocal Type Chart, C4 stands for middle C on the keyboard. If you're using a tamboura drone app, you'll be able to select the 3 or the 4 (referring to which octave you're singing to) from within the app.

Here are some likely areas where you'll find your sweet spot, based on your vocal type:

Bass—Around B♭2
Baritone—Around D3
Tenor—Around F3

Alto—Around B♭3
Mezzo Soprano—Around D4
Soprano—Around F4

Let your own experience be your guide. What feels right to you? Does your throat feel completely relaxed? Do you like the way your voice resonates in the particular key you're exploring? If the answer is yes, you've tuned in to your home base! Once you feel like you've got it, you may want to write down this significant insight about your own unique vocal sweet spot. Over the days and weeks that follow as you continue to explore your voice and the chanting practices in this book, you can return again and again to this musical home base. Keep in mind that it's also perfectly okay to shift your vocal sweet spot up or down a little as your singing journey unfolds. Stay present with the feelings in your body as you sing and let your experience show you the way.

Determining our vocal type through the techniques shared in this chapter and then utilizing this new insight about ourselves to discover our vocal sweet spot is not a mere musical exercise. Through our willingness to explore and learn about our own unique physical instrument through which we sing, speak, and express ourselves, we are learning more about who we are, and who we are not. Taking this journey of self-discovery through the healing act of singing is one of the greatest gifts we can give to our loved ones, our communities, our world, and ourselves.

Now that we've found our vocal home base, in the following chapter we'll dive deeper into the tools, techniques, and insights that will support us in allowing the flower of our voice to blossom fully and freely.

Chapter 5

The Yoga of Mindful Singing

Singing is like a celebration of oxygen.

—Björk

The human voice is truly the original musical instrument. Before there were drums or flutes or any of the other musical inventions that humans were inspired to create to accompany their singing, we had our voices. Over the centuries and across the globe, our diverse world cultures have found wildly different modes of singing to express the joys, sorrows, and experiences of life's journey. Whether it's the microtonal ululations of the Bulgarian women's choir, the prayerful monophonic style of Gregorian chant, the barbed-wire timbre of Bob Dylan, or the heavenly grandeur of a choir performing Bach's Mass in B Minor, every single singer among all those staggeringly diverse vocal styles— and every single human being as well, for that matter—shares one common characteristic: we are all honorary members of the Wind instrument family.

If you've ever attended one of those *Young Person's Guide to the Orchestra* performances that your local symphony puts on from time to time, you might recall being introduced to these four categories of musical instruments: the soaring Strings that include instruments like violins and cellos, the bright Brass with trumpets and trombones, the rhythmic Percussion with drums and cymbals, and, finally, the Winds or Woodwinds that include instruments such as flutes and saxophones. Although you and I may not have the smooth bamboo body of a bansuri flute or the shiny metal one of a saxophone, the flesh and bones of our physical instrument produces our singing voice in much the same way.

The Dance of the Breath

Essentially, a Wind instrument is one that uses air to make sound. While that description also applies to our friends in the Brass family, there's a distinction that sets the Wind instruments apart. Whereas trumpets, trombones, and the like create sound when the player's lips buzz together against a metal mouthpiece, in the Wind family the sound comes from the player's breath passing over an open surface—as with a flute—or over a thin wooden reed—as with a saxophone—producing the vibrations that create the sound of the instrument. Similarly, when we sing, the breath from our lungs passes over the thin membrane of our vocal cords (or more accurately, vocal folds) in our larynx, causing them to vibrate and produce sound. And although we could at least imagine a violinist or any other String instrument player holding her breath while still managing to serenade a room full of enchanted listeners (for a minute or so, anyway), when it comes to the Wind instruments, if there is no breath, there is no music. Period.

This dynamic dance of the breath is the life and soul of all singing, whether we're simply chanting a few *Oms* at the beginning of a yoga practice or we're about to belt out "One Day More" onstage in *Les Misérables*. Even though I'm guessing that most of you reading these pages might tend more toward the *Om* side of that spectrum, the same basic principles apply. Through the course of this chapter on the yoga of singing, we'll learn how to support, open, and nurture the instrument of our own unique body so that our true voice can blossom fully.

As we're learning about the mechanics of singing and how to support ourselves in letting our voices come forth with ease and freedom, keep in mind that—while on one hand we are simply developing our singing abilities—we are actually engaged in the deep soul work of healing, of singing ourselves more fully into being. Far from a mere tool of entertainment, our voice is a direct, living connection to the deepest parts of ourselves. Finding our true voice and releasing and expressing that voice can play a powerful role in finding and expressing our true selves.

> At the root of all power and motion, there is music and rhythm, the play of patterned frequencies against the matrix of time. We know that every particle in the physical universe takes its characteristics from the pitch and pattern and overtones of its particular frequencies, its singing. Before we make music, music makes us.
>
> —JOACHIM-ERNST BERENDT

Vocal Yoga

We'll begin the journey of finding our voice with a powerful practice called Breathing Through the Universe that I first learned from Daniel Comstock, a master voice teacher and the director for the Center for Attitudinal Healing & the Arts in Montana. A professional musician and conductor with a doctorate in musical arts, Daniel also brings three decades' worth of expertise in the transformational insights of "attitudinal healing" to his work as a voice teacher. His approach to singing deftly blends the most effective techniques for supporting and opening the voice while maximizing singing's potential as a powerful therapeutic tool for healing and self-actualization. As Daniel likes to say, "I don't really separate out personal support work in therapy from teaching people to sing. It's all the same to me."

Mindful of the fact that, as singers, we are truly a Wind instrument, we want to make sure that we are breathing fully and deeply. This next practice will help us to really open our chest and our lungs so that we can maximize our breath. More than that, it will attune us to our living connection with the energy of the Universe, allowing us to feel supported and filled by that energy. Before beginning the practice, you might find it helpful to do a few rounds of alternate nostril breathing (*nadi shodhana*) or any other kind of *pranayama* (yogic breathing) technique that you're familiar with.

As you move through this practice, allow yourself to become fully present, to inhabit your body with awareness and attention. Cultivate a strong sense of connection to the infinite energy of the Universe, letting it fill you from head to toe. When we sing from this place of connection, of fullness, we always have enough and we are at peace. Then, from this place of peace and presence, we give ourselves permission to sing. You might say to yourself, *I'm here right now in this body at this time. I have the right to do this and I deserve to feel good.* We give ourselves permission to be here and permission to manifest before we sing a single note.

Breathing Through the Universe

1. While standing with both feet rooting firmly into the earth, use your awareness to scan your body from your toes all the way up to the crown of your head. As your awareness scans over the length of your entire body, feel your life-energy and presence filling and embodying every inch of your physical form. Feel your body becoming activated, primed, and engaged through the power of your attention and awareness.

2. With an inhalation, slowly lift both hands up straight above and slightly in front of you with the palms facing forward. As you breathe in, imagine that your hands are gathering in the energy of the Universe. Sense that energy being drawn into your body, filling you with energy and support.

3. With an exhalation, the palms turn in toward the forehead and the hands slowly draw down toward your belly, continuing to gather the energy of the Universe. As you continue to exhale, imagine that you're sending the energy through your body, out your feet, and back down into the earth.

4. Repeat steps one to three for a few minutes, long enough to feel a sense of flowing balance between Yin and Yang, between receiving in and radiating out.

When you feel full and flowing, you can add the voice:

5. With your next inhalation, again slowly lift both hands up, gathering up the energy of the Universe to fill you with power and support.

6. Then, with your next exhalation, sing a descending "Ahhh" as you slowly draw your hands back down toward your belly. Feel that you are continuing to gather energy and support from the Universe—almost as if you are breathing in while singing out—sending the energy down through your body and out the soles of your feet.

7. Flow between steps five and six for as long as you'd like, cultivating a felt sense of balance between receiving the energy in and then sending it back out to the Universe.[12]

The Breathing Through the Universe practice is a beautiful starting point to open our voices. Through this practice, we can bring the Yin and Yang aspects of singing—gathering in what we need from the Universe, then sending the sound back out—into a flowing balance. This practice also helps us to consciously connect our physical body with the sound we're producing, bringing a kind of intentional integration to the entire singing experience.

> **The simplest way to think about breath support is to feel like you're breathing in while you're singing out.**
> —WILLIAM VENNARD

Discovering the Elixir Field

Having practiced the Breathing Through the Universe exercise for a few minutes to awaken the breath more fully, to bring more presence into our body, and to cultivate a sense of balanced flow with the energy of the Universe, we're ready to connect to our vocal support system. This is the essential root from which our voice can truly blossom.

In Taoism, martial arts, and Chinese medicine, this energy center is known as *Dan Tien*, which literally means "red field" but is sometimes poetically translated as "elixir field" or "sea of Chi." The Dan Tien is our body's center of gravity and is said to be the center of our physical and energy bodies as well. Situated in the lower belly, one-and-one-half thumb widths below the navel and two to three thumb widths inside the body, the Dan Tien is sometimes described as "the root of the Tree of Life." Whereas the heart serves the body by pumping blood, the Dan Tien is said to pump *Chi*, or energy. There are, according to the Taoist tradition, two other Dan Tien centers as well—one at the solar plexus and one between the eyebrows. But the lower Dan Tien, as it is sometimes called, is considered to be the foundation of breath and embodied awareness. This is the center from which our singing voice will arise.

The Dan Tien is located in a very particular spot in our anatomy, right at the bottom of the stomach area where the pubic region begins. If you place your hands right at this point and breathe in, you'll feel the tautness in your lower abdomen. If you breathe in a little more, you'll feel the tautness increase. Now, with your hands still over your lower abdomen, make a sound like an owl, "hoo hoo," but sweeping up and down in pitch. As you do this, you'll feel that tautness become active and the muscles in that region will go down and out a little bit.

To really get a basic feel for the lower abdominal muscles involved in supporting the voice, try this little exercise:

1. Sit down in a straight-back chair with your hands on the Dan Tien
2. Lean back in the chair a little bit
3. Now lift both feet up off the floor just a couple of inches

The musculature you feel activated in this little exercise is the same one that we use to support our voice when we sing. As another way of getting a sense of our abdominal support system, you can also lie down flat on the floor while lifting both legs up a few inches into the air.

Now that we have a general sense of where the Dan Tien is, we're going to take that insight and expand on it. In order for our voice to be fully supported, we want the expansion we just felt in the lower abdomen to circle all the way around the circumference of the body. We'll learn how to do this in a fun and easy little vocal gardening exercise called Finding Your Inner Flowerpot.

Letting the Flower of the Voice Blossom

I like to imagine that our singing voice is blossoming from our bodies like a kind of audible, vibrational flower. The actual sound that emerges from our mouths is like the blossoming petals of that flower, colorful and captivating, but it's the roots of the plant that support that blossom and give it life. The analogy of the flower is useful when we're cultivating our singing voice because, just like a flower, the voice can't fully blossom without the necessary root support system.

We've already gotten a general sense of where the voice finds its roots in the Dan Tien. Now let's do a simple exercise to expand that into an experience of how it feels to properly support our singing voice.

Finding Our Inner Flowerpot

1. Sitting or standing, begin with your hands over the Dan Tien as we had them in the last exercise.
2. Keeping your hands in line with the Dan Tien, place them on your belly, just below your rib cage with your middle fingers touching near the belly button.
3. Inhale fully and feel the walls of your diaphragm expand out against your hands as your lungs fill with air.
4. Exhale and feel how your diaphragm naturally shrinks as the air leaves your body. Do this a few times to get a feel for your natural diaphragmatic motion as you inhale and exhale.

Now we're going to engage our inner flowerpot:

5. Inhale again, feeling your diaphragm press into your hands.
6. As you exhale this time, use the diaphragmatic muscles to keep pressing your belly into your hands even as the air leaves your body. Try to get the sense that this outward expansion you're creating is extending in a complete circle around your body—front, back, and sides. This is the inner flowerpot.

7. Repeat steps five and six several times, really tuning in to how it feels to expand out in all directions, even as you are exhaling.

Now let's add the voice:

8. Inhale again, feeling your diaphragm press into your hands.
9. With your exhalation, sing "ah," "oh," or "ee" while still keeping the outward expansion of the diaphragm all the way around your body. As you sing, continue to expand out through your diaphragm, especially as you come to the end of your breath.
10. Repeat steps eight and nine for as long as you like, rotating between the different vowel sounds.

Once you're familiar with the practice, you can work on developing it further:

11. Inhale once more, feeling your diaphragm press into your hands.
12. This time on your exhalations, simply count out loud, "one, two, three, four, five," at the rate of one count per second, while still keeping the expansion of your diaphragm all the way around your body.
13. If you're able to maintain that expansion all the way up to the count of five, try moving on to counting up to ten, then fifteen, then twenty. Eventually, see if you can maintain your supported expansion all the way up to a count of thirty.

Finding Your Inner Flowerpot is a great way to tune in to your vocal support system. If you're new to singing or if you haven't explored the experience of vocal support, this exercise is a great way to get familiar with how it should feel in your body when you sing. As you're first learning the technique, it's a good idea to spend some quality time with the practice so that you can really build a solid foundation from which your voice can blossom. Once you're more familiar with the practice, you might try just doing four or five rounds before moving on to other things, just to make sure your vocal support system is engaged. Finally, if you happen to notice any tightness or tension in your throat during one of your singing or chanting sessions, this could be a reminder to check back in with your inner flowerpot to make sure you've still got that solid foundation activated every single time you sing.

....

Peace is the inner nature of humankind. If you find it within yourself, you will then find it everywhere.
—RAMANA MAHARSHI

....

A Few More Vocal Tips

The exercises and techniques we've already covered will prepare us to sing fully embodied, totally energized, and with proper vocal support. Now we'll learn a few little tricks to help open and release tension in some areas that you may not have even noticed before but that are essential to opening our voice. Kate Hart, a Grammy-nominated singer and vocal coach, shared these techniques with me.[13]

Tongue Yoga

There's more tension held in the back of the tongue than almost anywhere else in the body. We want to release this stuck energy so that our entire vocal apparatus can flow freely.

1. Using a clean handkerchief or a washcloth, gently take hold of the tip of your tongue with both of your hands.
2. Now gently but firmly pull your tongue up, down, and to either side.
3. Repeat step two a few more times.

This exercise will probably feel uncomfortable in the beginning because you're literally pulling the tension out. The tongue is obviously such an essential part of your singing and speaking and after releasing this tension you'll feel much more open and relaxed. The difference for most people is just huge! Often when I do this I feel the muscles in the back of my tongue gently "pop" and release, kind of like cracking a knuckle. It's an odd feeling but the benefits of this technique speak for themselves.

Another fabulous technique for releasing this stored tension in the back of the throat is a little move we'll borrow from yoga called Lion's Breath.

1. Stick your tongue out as far as you can, laying it as flat as you can on your chin.
2. With your tongue still extended, let out a nice, long "Ahh," feeling the tension leave your body.
3. Repeat steps one and two several times.

Happy Motorboat Exercise

Finally, you can try fluttering your lips together while singing any kind of sound you like while you do it, making a sound like a happy motorboat. If there's tension in the muscles of your face and mouth, you won't be able to get the flutter action, so this is a great way to get instant feedback about whether or not everything is properly relaxed.

Proper Care and Feeding of Your Voice

Let's return once more to our analogy of the voice being like a flower. It's impossible to overstate just how vital proper hydration really is to the health and longevity of our voice and, of course, to our overall health and well-being. For the flower of our voice to fully blossom, our vocal folds have to be kept moist so that they can move easily and vibrate freely. If you drink the recommended amount of eight eight-ounce glasses of water a day it will keep those vocal folds happy and hydrated. Next time you find your singing voice feeling less than 100 percent, just pause for a moment to drink a glass of water. When you return to singing, you'll probably feel a noticeable improvement in your voice.

In addition to good hydration, I'm also a big fan of drinking warm lemon water every morning. It's great for our overall health because it helps the body to detox naturally and it has lots of vitamin C. Most importantly for our voices, though, it helps clear away any thick, sticky buildup of mucus on the vocal folds. When we sing or speak, those vocal folds are rubbing against one another at a blinding speed of around one hundred to two hundred times a second. Fortunately, there's a natural coating of mucus on the vocal folds that allows them to move against one other gracefully, provided that the coating is thin and slippery, kind of like motor oil in the engine of a car. If that coating gets gunked up and sticky, however, the vocal folds can't move smoothly and our voice isn't going to feel right. Besides, in the same way that old, thick, sticky oil will make a car engine run rough and eventually damage it, over time we can injure the delicate tissue of the vocal folds by not clearing out the old sticky stuff that might be clogging them up.

To keep your vocal folds healthy, flowing, and strong I recommend starting your day with a nice cup of warm lemon water. Just squeeze the juice from half a lemon into about six ounces of warm water and enjoy. This simple little regimen will do wonders for your voice and will keep those all-important vocal folds purring like a well-tuned engine.

Fertilizing the Soil

We'll finish this chapter on the yoga of singing with a helpful little checklist called "The Three Priorities" that we can refer to anytime we want to prepare ourselves to sing. In the same way that an athlete or a runner will warm up before jumping into action—warming up the muscles so that they're primed, protected from injury, and working at their best—singing is a dynamic activity that we are well served to prepare for in breath, body, heart, and mind. This simple yet essential three-step checklist is another little gem from Daniel Comstock, and it's an incredibly effective way to quickly engage all the singing principles and techniques we learned in the vocal yoga section.

The Three Priorities

1. Embodying Your Instrument

When we sing, our body, heart, and mind *become* our musical instrument. So, having the felt sense of fully inhabiting ourselves—in body, emotion, and thought—is the most important starting point. Begin by infusing your entire body with an activating awareness, wrapping your body in *prana* (the vital life force) to enliven and engage every part of you from head to toe. This is the concept of "animated posture," the felt sense that your entire body is poised as though you're about to move. Even when we're sitting cross-legged on the floor, we put as much attention on our whole body as we can, cultivating the sense that the body is fully active and ready to move. If we're standing, our body feels engaged from head to toe, as if we're poised to jump to the back of the room. This is not about creating tension in the body but, rather, engagement and embodiment. We now know that our whole body works as a unit, so if we turn off one part of our body, the rest of our body follows suit and does some kind of turning off in response. In the same way, if you get tense or grip in one part of your body, the rest of your body responds in kind.

This first step of Embodying Your Instrument means we are preparing our instrument by bringing an engaged, active presence into the here and now of our physical body. If we're doing it right, it can feel like we're ready to fly. Then, to bring the heart and mind into alignment as well, we give ourselves permission to sing. We might say to ourselves, "I'm here right now in this body at this time.

I have the right to do this and I deserve to feel good."
We give ourselves permission to be here and permission
to manifest before we sing a single note. We fully arrive
physically, emotionally, and mentally to the experience of
opening our voice.

2. Yawning Breath

If you notice, anytime we yawn we always go down
into an abdominal breath and it always engages the
Dan Tien. We may not be aware of it, though, because
our culture often encourages us to be turned off from
the waist down. The Yawning Breath practice is a great
way to quickly connect to this root of energetic power.
The second benefit of the Yawning Breath is that it will
help us to open up our physical instruments in order to
increase the sound of the voice and to make that sound
more pleasing. We'll do this by opening up our own
resonating space within the instrument of our physical
body.

When you do the Yawning Breath, try to make it as
much like an actual yawn as possible. Open your mouth
wide and feel your jaw gently stretching. If you're doing
it right, you'll feel your voice box (the Adam's apple)
moving down if you place one hand on your throat.

There are three components to the Yawning Breath:

+ Prepare your instrument by opening and relaxing
  your mouth and throat. Connect with your body,
  which is already engaged and activated from step one.
+ Take a yawning, abdominal breath. Feel it engaging
  the Dan Tien.

+ Sense your body filling with the energy of the
Universe. Feel that you have all the energy you need
for whatever you're about to sing.

3. Supported Sigh

When we sigh, our vocal folds are relaxed and there's
a natural equilibrium between the gently exhaling air and
the resistance of the vocal folds. The special relaxed and
balanced quality of a sigh creates a consistent flowing
sound in the voice. Practicing the Supported Sigh offers
a great way to get familiar with how it feels to sing with
the vocal folds relaxed.

+ As you exhale, sigh "Ahhh" in a soft, open voice for
four or five seconds.
+ As you sustain the "Ahhh," engage your inner
flowerpot, creating support for your voice by
expanding out in the Dan Tien and lower back.
Through this expansion, feel as if you're breathing in
as you're singing out.
+ Strive to make the sound consistent, with no breaks.

Repeat these three steps eight to ten times.

Before beginning any singing or chanting session, you can go
through the above "Three Priorities" to prepare the ground for
the flower of your voice to blossom. As you get more and more
familiar with the qualities described in this handy vocal checklist,
as well as those from the earlier exercises, you'll embody these
qualities in your own singing style naturally. By building a solid
foundation with these powerful vocal techniques, you'll find that
over time they'll become second nature to you.

You might also find that these vocal insights are coming into play for you in the midst of your daily life—the next time you're singing in your car or in your shower, for instance, or perhaps at a kirtan. Anytime at all that you happen to open your mouth to sing, these principles of mindful singing are there for you to draw on for support and inspiration. You might even find that the insights from these practices give you a new and palpable sense of connection, presence, and energetic support simply by bringing them to mind as you're speaking with a friend or family member, going about your day, or even just taking in a natural breath.

You can greatly enhance this empowering experience by finding just a few minutes every day to give yourself the gift of mindful singing. After we conclude this portion of the book, we'll journey on to Part Two: Music and Mantras, and Part Three: Songbook for the Soul, where we'll discover a wealth of inspiring opportunities to explore mindful singing, mantra, and chanting in our daily lives. Before we embark on the next part of our singing adventure, however, we'll learn a simple yet powerful practice that we can begin right now to experience the life-enhancing benefits of mindful singing for ourselves. My hope is that this will become an inspiring daily practice for you to energize and fuel your voyage through the next parts of the book.

An Experience of Mindful Singing:
The 5-Minute *Om*

Find a comfortable, quiet spot where you won't be disturbed for at least the next five minutes or so. You might find it helpful to do this singing practice at the same time every day—perhaps first thing in the morning to mindfully gather your energy in preparation for the day ahead, or in the evening as a way to calm and center yourself to settle down for a restful night. In addition, you can use this powerful practice as needed anytime you'd like to clear your energy, relieve stress or anxiety, center yourself in preparation for an important meeting or event, or even as a means of sending energetic healing and positive intentions to others.

When first learning the 5-Minute *Om*, you can simply sing along with the audio link below. Once you're familiar with the practice, though, you might want to explore a different musical key to sing in based on your own vocal sweet spot. For this, you'll want to support yourself with the sound of a musical drone from a tamboura app as we discussed in the "Drone Zone" chapter or from a harmonium or keyboard of your choice.

The 5-Minute *Om* practice follows the magical six-breaths-per-minute-style of singing that we learned about in the "Science of Singing" chapter. Since each *Om* we sing will sustain for about eight seconds, we'll want to make sure that we're tapping into the breathing and support techniques we learned earlier in this chapter. Before beginning, you might choose to warm up by going through the "Three Priorities" checklist: Embodying Your Instrument, Yawning Breath, and Supported Sigh. Alternatively, you might choose to do a few rounds of the Breathing Through the Universe exercise to prepare to sing. If time is short and you want to jump right into the practice, simply take three full inhalations and exhalations, filling your body with breath and energy before you sing.

When you're ready to begin, play the 5-Minute *Om* audio link:

5-Minute *Om*: GirishMusic.com/BookAudio

As you're enjoying the 5-Minute *Om* practice, remember and engage the principles of mindful singing that we've learned together. Tune in to the energetic sense of being supported and filled by the Universe as you sing. Give yourself permission to be here fully in this practice, to express yourself through your own voice. Connect with a strong sense of vocal support by engaging your inner flowerpot as you sing. Feel how your voice connects you with life and with the world around you. If feelings or emotions arise during your practice, allow your voice to release and express them, clearing any blocked energy within you.

At the end of the 5-Minute *Om* practice, you might find that you're naturally inspired to sit a while longer, enjoying the new sense of peace and clarity. Feel free to immerse yourself in this experience for as long as you choose, perhaps using this opportunity to set new intentions, seek insights or guidance, or simply offer gratitude. When you're ready to conclude the practice, you may wish to place your hands on your heart, knowing that you carry the healing energies of this experience with you as you go on with your day.

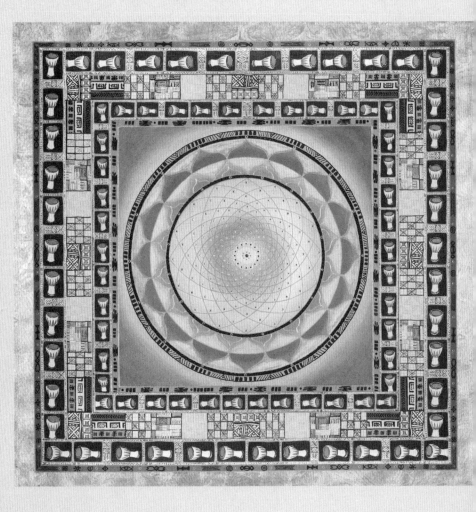

~~~

PART TWO

Music and Mantras

Chapter 6

My Adventure from Jazz Club to Ashram

Open the door and step out. The path will become visible. Once on the way, you will meet other wayfarers who will advise and guide you. Your job is to muster whatever strength you have to get underway. Thereafter, help is assured.

—Sri Anandamayi Ma

For as long as I can remember, I've felt deeply drawn to a life of music. By the time I was eight years old, I'd been tapping and banging out rhythms on anything I could get my hands on long enough for my parents to realize that my endless urge to drum was definitely going to outlast the upholstery on our car seats. So, that Christmas they gave me my very first instrument—a sparkly red Ludwig snare drum—with an understanding that I would kindly reserve my rhythmic enthusiasm solely for my new drum, and henceforth renounce my percussive assault upon every available surface.

Well, that was the plan, anyway.

What happened instead was that my little red snare became my gateway into the wide world of percussion instruments. It's just like that children's book *If You Give a Mouse a Cookie*, except it's called *If You Give a Kid a Snare Drum*. Because, as far as I was concerned, once you hear the pop of that snare, you've just got to have that low thump of a bass drum to go with it. And once you've got that snare and bass combo going, you know you've got to have some sweet tom-tom action so you can get your Ringo Starr on. And once you're grooving along with those toms in full effect like "Tomorrow Never Knows," you've just got to put the icing on the cake with some scintillating cymbal crashes.

By the time I got to junior high, I was rocking a full drum set—Ludwigs with natural blond wood shells and Zildjian cymbals all around. In the meantime, I'd been taking weekly drum lessons since I was eight, but hadn't really ventured outside the performance space of my downstairs den or my friend's garage. That all changed in eighth grade.

My best friend, Mark, and I played in the talent show that year, with him on guitar and me on those blond Ludwig drums. I'm not even totally sure what song we played. I'd like to imagine it sounded like a junior high version of the Black Keys, but what I *can* remember is the thrill of hearing the auditorium full of our classmates bursting into raucous applause. This new experience of connecting with my peers through the medium of music made a powerful and lasting impression on me. I felt seen and appreciated in a way I never had before. From that point on, I wasn't just another kid: I was a musician.

All through high school and college, music was my passion, my practice, and by the time I got to University of Tennessee, Knoxville—my profession. I played in every imaginable musical ensemble in high school: jazz band, orchestra, percussion ensemble, marching band—playing every percussion instrument known to man in every conceivable style of music. By the time I got to college, I was still musically multitasking with four or five different ensembles at any given time, but right from that first year at UT I was venturing out to play gigs as a professional drummer.

In those days, there was a thriving live music scene flourishing in Knoxville's Old City. Originally built by Irish immigrants who came to Knoxville to help lay the railroad in the 1850s, this funky, urban neighborhood on the northeast side of town had rebounded from its "raucous, vice-ridden" past after a revitalization effort in the 1990s sparked a renaissance of sorts. There was a distinct New Orleans flare in the Old City, with jazz clubs on every corner. On any given Friday or Saturday night, there was a good chance you'd see me behind the drums at Annie's, a jazz club run by a vivacious Brit named Annie DeLisle, who happened to be novelist Cormac McCarthy's ex-wife.

As much as I was immersed in the world of jazz drumming during those college years, I have to say that this wasn't born out of some burning passion for jazz on my part. I mean, as a style of music I enjoyed jazz, but I definitely was not among the die-hards who walked the halls of the UT music department with me. My personal tastes in music, even in those days, ventured out into an eclectic territory of singer/songwriter, alternative/folk pop, and world music that my jazzhead friends really had no use for. But what inspired me to be so devoted to practicing and performing jazz in those days—beyond the fact that jazz was where the paying gigs were—was my recognition that jazz was arguably the pinnacle of musical expression, technique, and artistry for a drummer. The intricacies and variations of rhythm that a jazz drummer is called upon to master are vast. I reasoned that, even if jazz wasn't my true love in terms of musical styles, if I could play jazz, I could play anything.

Fortunately for me, my college years at UT happened to coincide with a golden era in its music department. Under the direction of legendary instructor and saxophonist Jerry Coker, the jazz program at that time was bustling with motivated and devoted kids like me who had fire in their bellies to become great musicians. We were drawn there by the school's reputation for excellence and we weren't disappointed. I had the great fortune to study with Keith Brown, drum teacher extraordinaire, who was not only a patient and expert instructor but also truly cared for his students and was deeply devoted to our growth and success as musicians. I would spend the week practicing long hours every day to prepare for my weekly lessons. Knowing how much Keith believed in and encouraged my abilities, it was important to me that I made him proud every time I sat in front of him to play.

The real proving ground for all the skills and techniques that I learned in those weekly lessons with Keith, however, was out in the classroom of live performance. Whatever funky drum groove or flashy fill or fancy new technique he had taught me in my lessons had to be integrated somehow into actual music, otherwise it was just a kind of musical unicorn that didn't exist in the real world. Luckily, I had no shortage of opportunities to figure out how all those techniques could be transformed into real, live music. Two or three nights a week I'd be out performing somewhere, playing every conceivable style of music from big band swing to straight-ahead jazz to funk to fusion to rock to Motown and Top 40. As a professional drummer, I wanted to learn every style of music I might be called upon to play. And even though I wasn't quite sure yet exactly where my musical destiny was taking me, I knew at least this way I'd have all my stylistic bases covered.

As it turned out, my destiny did come calling in those days playing jazz at Annie's in the Old City. It came in the form of a spiritual experience masquerading as just an ordinary night on the bandstand.

My Jazz Communion

If someone asked me to summarize the entire musical idiom of jazz in just one word, I'd probably have to say "improvisation." If you were to stroll down to the Blue Note club in NYC tonight, perhaps you'd be greeted by the sounds of a little trio—piano, bass, and drums—playing through their set of jazz standards like "Autumn Leaves," "Satin Doll," or "Take the 'A' Train." And imagine for a moment that you're walking through the doors of the Blue Note not as you but as, say, an interstellar musician visiting from a galaxy far, far away in which there was no such thing as jazz. The first thing your highly attuned audio-sensing organs would notice is that, in fact, these guys are mostly just making this stuff up on the fly. Yes, they'll play the recognizable, composed melody of the tune (the "head") at the beginning and again at the end, but everything else that happens during the sprawling, dynamic musical free-for-all in between—*they are making that shit up!* This is improvisation, the heart and soul of jazz music.

Now, truth be told, even though jazz improvisation is incredibly creative and spontaneous, it doesn't usually result in complete tonal anarchy (except when it does) because the musicians are actually still following the same chord progression (or "changes") throughout the entire song. So, even though we may not hear the pianist playing the familiar melody of, say, "The Girl from Ipanema" in the middle of the song during his solo, if you were to sing that melody out loud during that solo, you'd notice that the chords the band is playing still fit with it. In other words, the creativity and the freedom exist within or on top of a musical framework (or "form")—typically the progression of chords, the number of bars (or "measures"), and the tempo.

Even so, that form is more like a blueprint than a painting or a photograph, because it leaves a great deal open to the interpretation and creativity of the musicians. Or you might imagine the form as being a bit like an X-ray of someone's body: you can see that there's a head here and arms there and legs down there, but that X-ray won't tell you anything about eye color, hair color, skin tone, or what mood the owner of those bones might happen to be in. In the same way, the form leaves all of those nuanced details of the song open to interpretation. The musicians flesh out the complete picture, with all its subtleties and revelations, in the moment through improvisation.

At this point, you certainly might know more about jazz than you did a couple of paragraphs ago and possibly even more than you really care to, but this preamble sets us up for what comes next. The experience I want to share unfolded in the context of this dynamic world of controlled chaos, of freedom within form, in which jazz improvisation lives and breathes. There's often an edge-of-your-seat quality to playing live jazz because you're aware that, should inspiration strike, the music could turn suddenly in unexpected ways, taking the band along with it. It might sound strange to speak of music as a living thing like that, capable of taking able-bodied young musicians by surprise, but it's true and it happens all the time.

There were countless moments onstage playing with whatever group I happened to be joining that night, where—with no prearranged plan to do so and with no words or cues exchanged between the members of the band—we all instantly and simultaneously *knew* how and where to make a quantum leap together so that our musical caterpillar suddenly transformed and took flight as a butterfly. This is not hyperbole. There was no linear, predictable path from point A to point B, from the way we *had* been playing the song to this entirely new interpretation of the very same song. Maybe it was a sudden shift in the groove or feel, or perhaps a dramatic change in dynamics, but whatever the nature of the quantum musical shift, each and every member of the ensemble seemed to be in the loop, as if we'd each received an instantaneous "Chi-mail" directly to our brains alerting us to our new musical game plan.

These moments of jazz communion were not some rare, exotic experience; they were just the hallmark of a "good gig." If we were really listening to one another, if we had our hearts, minds, and souls in the music, then, more often than not, the magic would strike at least once during the night. And even though this experience was familiar, that didn't make it any less miraculous to me. In fact, every time it happened, I'd feel an exuberant joy sweeping over me, like I was cresting the hill on some giant roller coaster. It was so much more than just good music to me; it was the profound joy of knowing, of experiencing for myself directly and without a doubt, that I was somehow connected with my bandmates, with everyone in the audience, with Life itself.

Over the course of my time at UT, I relished those experiences of musical communion and, more than that, found myself changed by them. Actually feeling that sense of connection, that oneness, was inspiring and intriguing to me in a way that kindled my lifelong curiosity about spiritual life. I had never been religious in a traditional way, but I was always interested in the possibility of a spiritual realm, even though I hadn't really experienced it for myself before. Now, for the first time, I was having these moments of undeniable connection that felt authentically spiritual to me. My worldview began to shift on its axis because I genuinely believed that these glimpses of oneness proved beyond a doubt there really was a spiritual dimension to life. Once that became real for me, experiencing that dimension as fully and as often as I could became my new passion.

It may have been this newly awakened enthusiasm for all things spiritual or maybe it was just that it fulfilled some liberal arts credits toward my major in English and creative writing, but during my second year at UT, I signed up for a course in the philosophy department on comparative world religions. In hindsight, it's clear when thinking back on the class syllabus and the sequence of world spiritual philosophies we progressed through that I can see my own personal spiritual journey there mapped out in broad strokes.

As the class moved from one world religion and philosophy to another, from the dreary landscape of Marxism to the stained-glass world of Christianity and Judaism, the baton was eventually passed from Jesus to Buddha. Our class ventured back in time by about six centuries prior to the birth of Christianity and into the unfamiliar realm of Buddhism. Even so, I noticed that there were certain traits that Buddhism shared with the Christian faith that I had grown up with in the Presbyterian Church. There was the common theme of "do unto others" morality and ethics, expressed in Buddhism through the teachings of loving-kindness, compassion, and karma (what you reap is what you sow). There was the fact that both traditions revolve around a central spiritual figure, in the form of Jesus or Buddha. However, beyond these and a few other common threads, I discovered that at the heart of Buddhism there was a radically different and powerfully enticing core concept. Buddhism teaches that the goal of the spiritual path is not a heavenly reward in the afterlife but, rather, a direct spiritual experience here and now in this very life.

New words like *enlightenment, nirvana,* and *satori* drifted into my ears like enchanting music from some other dimension. As our professor listed the qualities and characteristics of the experience of *nirvana* (bliss, wisdom, love, union with the Divine) something switched on inside of me. People were actually having this experience that my professor was describing to us, possibly right at that very moment, real human beings like you and me. And it wasn't just one enlightened guy, it was lots of men and women throughout the ages who had successfully reached the goal. If they could have this experience, that meant that I could, too.

The import of this realization dawned gradually but steadily over the next several months. Meanwhile, our class journeyed onward to the spiritual world of Hinduism, with its radiant constellations of Deities like Shiva, Durga, Hanuman, Krishna, Lakshmi, and Saraswati. I wondered how an ordinary Hindu could be expected to keep track of all these gods and goddesses. However, I soon learned that, contrary to my mistaken understanding of that ancient spiritual tradition, Hinduism isn't actually a polytheistic religion at all. In fact, Hinduism is possibly the ultimate monotheistic spiritual tradition. Not only are all the gods and goddesses seen as simply manifestations of the one, all-encompassing Divinity, but everything else is as well—all living beings, nature, and the Universe. And, not to be outdone, Hinduism also has its version of the enlightenment experience: *samadhi.*

It was there while our intrepid class explored the nuances of

Hinduism that I was first introduced to the practice of mantra and chanting. I remember seeing black-and-white photographs of yogis in our course textbook, eyes closed in meditation, *japa mala* (rosary) beads in hand. Judging from the looks on their faces, these yogis were most definitely deep in some exalted state. I wondered, *Is this what samadhi looks like?* Seeing them, even in a photograph, made the possibility of genuine direct spiritual experience tantalizingly real for me. I knew that I had tasted little glimpses of oneness in my communion experiences through music. But as electrifying and transforming as those glimpses had been, they were brief and unpredictable. I was yearning for more.

By the end of that semester, I left that class a different person than the one who had walked in that very first day. Now I understood that these little tastes of spiritual experience that I'd found through music were familiar territory for these enlightened beings called yogis, sadhus, lamas, monks, and saints. I knew that there was not just one but many spiritual traditions, and they had already blazed a path, a system of practices that people just like me had followed to the goal of direct and genuine spiritual experience. I left that class awake and alive to the prospect that I could seek out and find these living spiritual traditions, even there in Tennessee.

I returned to my college routine—attending classes during the week, playing gigs on the weekend—but in the midst of that familiar schedule, I was actually beginning my newfound quest. My eyes were keenly on the lookout for any mention of the words *yoga*, *mantra*, or *meditation*. I began reading any books on the subject I could get my hands on, and I found a group that met every Thursday night called SER, or Spiritual Enlightenment Research.

Theresa, one of the leaders of the group, was a student of Yogi Bhajan's and she led me in my very first yoga class during one of our many Thursday-night sessions. I was grateful to find that there were elders like Theresa in my community, people who discovered the spiritual path decades before me and were ready and willing to share their insights and experience. She and the other three leaders in the group would take turns guiding our Thursday sessions, each from their own unique perspective and tradition.

My favorite nights were the ones in which we learned meditation, pranayama, yoga *asanas* (physical postures), and mantra. Every session culminated with a spiritual discourse and group discussion, facilitated by that week's leader. Our minds, hearts, and spirits were nourished by the teachings and the practices, and the spices of the yogi tea that Theresa always kept on tap warmed our bellies. Having found a sense of spiritual community in this group, I rarely missed a Thursday meeting. With the diverse array of traditions and perspectives that the leaders presented, SER was really a kind of spiritual banquet where us newbies to the path could taste and sample all the rich flavors that the various traditions had to offer. For me, though, it was becoming more and more apparent that I was being called to the path of meditation and mantra.

As a junior in college then with a wide-ranging passion for music, I'd heard recordings of mantras here and there, and I'd definitely felt a certain captivating and calming quality from them. That feeling inspired me to integrate mantra music into the soundtrack of my college life—a diverse mix that included John Coltrane, Miles Davis, Naná Vasconcelos, R.E.M., and Elvis Costello, alongside the symphonies of Gustav Mahler. As broad as my musical tastes were, there was something truly unique about mantra music that exerted a kind of gravitational pull, urging me to go deeper and discover more. I was meditating with the group every Thursday and had even begun a daily yoga asana practice at home, often with the sounds of my favorite mantra recording playing in the background. Still, I yearned to go deeper. I knew that if I wanted to truly explore the tradition of yoga and mantra in depth, I couldn't do it by reading about it in books and by trying to replicate the practices I'd read about in my bedroom. So, I turned my attention to a new possibility. Having already discovered for myself that there were indeed spiritual elders right there in my own community who were willing and able to share their wisdom, I opened myself to the prospect that I might also find someone who had actually reached the goal of the spiritual path—a living, enlightened being—right there in Tennessee.

Paradise in the Smoky Mountains

Around that time, a classified ad in the back of *Yoga Journal* magazine caught my eye. It read, "Paradise with MahaShakti Yoga Master." The area code for the phone number listed in the ad was 615, the same as mine. Intrigued and excited, I called and got the address and set a date and time when I could make the one-hour drive out to the foothills of the Smoky Mountains where the *ashram* (spiritual retreat) was located. A few days later when I finally made my first pilgrimage there, traffic was bad and I was running late. The sun had set by the time I rolled in and I could already hear music and voices wafting out from the main building as I approached, a sure sign that the evening program was already under way. Excited but a little apprehensive about walking in late, I resolved that I hadn't sought out this opportunity and traveled all this way just to turn around and head home, so I followed the sound of the music and made my way up the front steps.

The beauty of the scene that greeted me there as I opened the front door was enhanced by the intoxicating sound of voices chanting in unison and the sweet tones of the harmonium and tamboura. The vibrations of the instruments and the chanting seemed to create a kind of subtle energy field that permeated the space with a palpable presence. I removed my shoes and entered the shrine room for the very first time. As I began to carefully navigate my way between the two dozen or so people sitting cross-legged on the floor, I had the distinct sensation that I was moving through water or some other invisible substance that seemed to thicken the air around me.

It was like the sensation we get sometimes in dreams when we suddenly find gravity a much more formidable force than in waking life and simply walking becomes a slow-motion struggle to get from here to there. Besides, the room was illuminated only by the soft golden glow emanating from the oil lamps on the shrine. Moving slowly and cautiously was my best course of action since I really did not want to commemorate my maiden visit to the ashram by stepping on someone's foot. Eventually, though, I managed to find my way to an empty space on the floor and gratefully took my seat alongside the rest of the group, facing as they were in the direction of a beautiful altar that stretched from ceiling to floor.

Oil lamps flickered on the marble tiers of the shrine, illuminating several *murtis* (statues) of Hindu Deities framed against a backdrop of bright red and gold Indian silk designs. The walls around the room were decorated with life-sized portraits of yogis and saints, as well as images of the Hindu Deities—Durga on her lion and Shiva, eyes half closed in meditation. The sweet-smelling scent of an unfamiliar incense drifted across the room and I breathed in the tantalizing fragrance deeply.

I found myself swaying gently in my seat, all of my senses drinking in the fullness of this moment. The energetic and emotional impact of this first chanting experience was so rich and powerful for me, although I honestly had no idea at all what these people were singing or what it was supposed to mean. I remember trying to follow along in a chant book that someone handed to me, but the strange words on the page didn't seem to match the sounds I was hearing, so I just put the book down and listened. I closed my eyes and let the rhythmic flow of the voices and the exotic sounds of the instruments wash over me. My heart fluttered and raced, as if thrilled by the presence of some long-sought mystery finally revealed. Somehow, the vibrations of the chanting conveyed everything I needed to receive, even though whatever was happening was beyond the reach of my rational mind.

At the center of the sacred festivities unfolding there in the shrine room that night sat Shankaracharya Swami, playing the harmonium and leading the group in chanting. He was positioned right alongside the altar and I could see by the shimmering light from the oil lamps that he was dressed all in red, even the little wool cap that he wore. After twenty minutes or so, the chanting came to an end and Shankaracharya began to speak while the group sat in receptive meditative silence. For me, hearing the spiritual wisdom I'd been trying to find in books actually embodied and expressed through the words of a living teacher sitting right in front of me was exhilarating and a little otherworldly. I had to occasionally remind myself that I was still in Tennessee, just an hour from school, and not in some yogi's mountain hermitage in India. But there I was.

This moment marked a dramatic turn in the course of my life.

I began to visit the ashram as often as I could in between classes and gigs. It was clear to me that my search had led me to an authentic spiritual guide and the rarefied environment of a living yogic tradition. I had found exactly what I was looking for. Less than a year after my first visit, just one month after graduating from college, I became a full-time resident of the ashram. For the next five years, I immersed myself completely in a monastic life of mantra, meditation, and the wisdom teachings embodied by Shankaracharya and the Tantric lineage he represents.

I came to the ashram as a fervent young seeker, full of questions about spiritual life. I've heard it said that a great mentor or teacher doesn't merely provide answers to your questions, he or she gives you the tools you need to answer those questions for yourself. This is precisely the kind of teacher that Shankaracharya was for me and the other fortunate souls who've experienced his wise and loving guidance.

Tabla with a Twist

There's one final element in this part of the story of my musical adventure that I'd like to share. It's absolutely clear to me what a significant role drumming and music played not only in shaping the course of my life, but in kindling the fire in me that led me to the ashram and to immerse myself in spiritual life at such a young age. Yet, once I had reached this spiritual destination, once this radically new phase of my life had begun, I found that playing music—my lifelong passion—abruptly began to lose its luster for me.

During the better part of that first year at the ashram, even though I was a full-time resident I would still go out most week-ends to play drums back in Knoxville. I'd return to Annie's jazz club to play the same music with the same bands, but something was different. Those magical moments of jazz communion would strike, just like always, and each and every one of us in the band would revel in that shared experience of musical oneness. Yet, I began to notice that, for the most part, the magic of our experience existed only within the energetic bubble of the stage. What felt to me and the other players like thrilling moments of shared human connection was just background music for most members of the audience. They weren't *in it* with us. Granted, Annie's was a supper club. People came to eat, drink, and socialize. They weren't expected to sit in rapt attention to the live music at all times. Still, there was a sense of disconnection that felt disheartening to me, as if the experience was somehow incomplete.

The truth is, the music at Annie's hadn't changed, I had. At the ashram, I had been introduced to a whole new musical experience, one in which every single person in the room—whether playing an instrument or not—was in that energetic bubble, sharing in the joy and connection of the music. Every morning and night we would chant together, singing Sanskrit hymns, mantras, or call-and-response kirtan. The music was simple and heartfelt, with none of the intricacies or virtuosity of jazz. But what the chanting lacked in musical technique, it more than made up for in soul and an ability to generate these moments of ecstatic communion, which the entire group shared as one.

Coming into the ashram community as a professional drummer, I was quickly enlisted to learn to play the tablas to accompany the chanting. I'd never heard a percussion instrument that sounded anything like this before, with seemingly infinite variations of hypnotic tones arising from just two little drums. Having a lifetime of percussion experience under my belt, I felt pretty confident that I could find my way around the tablas without too much trouble. I quickly discovered, though, that these drums are really in a world of their own, both in terms of the technique it takes to get a proper sound out of them as well as the distinct and unfamiliar rhythms that are the hallmark of the Indian classical music tradition from which tablas emerge. When I first began playing, I failed miserably at both. I remember Shankaracharya complaining after a certain kirtan that the way I was playing "sounded like a Bossa Nova or something." He was right, actually. I was so steeped in the rhythms of jazz and Western music, my ears hadn't quite tuned in yet to the subtleties of these new Indian rhythms. Humbled, I decided to embrace the rather daunting challenge of learning the centuries-old art of playing the tablas.

My exotic percussion adventure was just getting under way during the same period in which I was finding myself so disheartened with playing jazz. My weekend gigs back in the city started to feel more and more like a distraction that were taking me away from what I really wanted to be doing—immersing myself in mantra practice and chanting. At the ashram, the tablas were my constant companion. I'd have my hands on the drums as much as I could in between the morning and evening programs and whatever work I was called upon to do during the day. I was motivated by a powerful desire to finally figure these things out so that I could rock our ashram chanting in proper Indian style. Even my small steps of progress felt satisfying and rewarding, and every night in the evening program I'd excitedly take to the drums again, hoping to serve and inspire the chanting to the best of my abilities.

It was around that time, when I was finally able to hold down a respectable tabla part for the kirtans—one that didn't sound like a Bossa Nova anymore—that I shocked myself and everyone else who knew me with a dramatic decision. Just nine months into my new life at the ashram, I announced to my bandmates that I wouldn't be playing gigs anymore. Shortly after that, I sold my fancy Sonor drum set. After more than fifteen years of passionate dedication, the life path and career of music as I had known it seemed to be over for me. My musician friends tried to talk me out of it. My parents, who had supported my musical journey from the very beginning, were in disbelief. And even though part of me felt sad to think that I was walking away for good from a life of music, there was a deep knowing in me that it was time for me to offer it up, to let it go. The joy and connection I was finding through mantra and chanting, especially now that tablas were part of the package, gave me the best of what I'd found in music before, but in much greater measure. At that moment, anyway, I fully expected that I'd happily live out my life as a tabla-playing monk deep in the mountains of Tennessee. But it seems that the spirit of music had other plans for me.

The summer of my fourth year at the ashram found me driving my parents' bright yellow VW Bug on a nonstop, thirteen-hour pilgrimage from the Smoky Mountains of Tennessee to the Catskills of New York. My drive was fueled by the sound of mantras blasting from the car speakers and the sweet smell of nag champa incense billowing out of the open car windows. My destination was a sacred music and meditation retreat led by spiritual teacher and musician Bob Kindler, known to his students as "Babaji." His albums, which feature contemporary renditions of mantra music, were in heavy rotation on the ashram stereo and had become a personal favorite of mine. I had started up a correspondence with him, telling him of my affinity for his music and about my burgeoning tabla skills. When he presented me with the opportunity to not only attend the retreat but to actually play tablas for him there, I was over the moon. In the backseat of the car, my tablas bounced along excitedly with me as I made my way to New York for the retreat with as few stops as humanly possibly.

The week that unfolded there in the Catskills with Babaji and the community of students who came to learn, meditate, and chant with him was a revelation for me. In the teachings and tradition that Babaji embodied I found equal parts spiritual wisdom and musical artistry. I did the best I could on the tablas to accompany his beautiful mantra music, which was far more intricate and diverse than the style of kirtan I had been familiar with. As far as I had come in my years of practicing tabla, it was clear that I still had a long way to go.

After a week of sacred music, mantra, and meditation in the Catskills, I was renewed, grateful, and inspired. Babaji's parting words to me were, "Go home and practice tablas for a year, then come and play with me." To hear these words from a teacher and artist whom I admired greatly filled me with unbelievable joy and inspiration. His invitation would reverberate in my mind and heart over the course of the year that followed. The seed had been planted. It was only a matter of time before it blossomed.

By the end of that next year, I had reached another turning point. After five years of living the monastic life of a yogi, I found that my love and passion for music had reawakened, but in a completely transformed state. Through years of experiencing group chanting at the ashram and listening to the recordings of artists like Babaji and his group Jai Ma Music, I began to see the possibility of a whole new expression of music, one in which everyone listening could join in the joyful experience of connection and communion. This new mantra-based form of sacred music was a blending of my two great passions: the power of mantra and the beauty of music. Besides, Babaji was not only a world-class cellist and composer, he was also an authentic spiritual guide, steeped in the wisdom tradition of Vedanta. His illustrious lineage traces directly back to the great Indian saint Sri Ramakrishna.

Realizing that I could continue to immerse myself in a life of meditation, mantra, and yogic wisdom while at the same time embarking on my journey into this new world of sacred music, playing tablas by his side at events all around the country, I left the ashram that December to join Babaji in Hawaii. I took initiation and began my studies with him, attending retreats and classes at his centers in Hawaii, Portland, and San Francisco after joining him and a small group for my maiden pilgrimage to India. For the next six years I immersed myself in the teachings and practices of Babaji's lineage, while also playing tablas with him for sacred music concerts across the United States. During this time, I found myself growing tremendously in both my spiritual and musical life through Babaji's wise and loving guidance.

Having returned to drumming through this new incarnation of sacred music, here is where this part of my musical journey comes full circle. Inspired by the level of musicianship that Babaji's music called me to, I decided to enroll in tabla classes at the Ali Akbar College of Music in Marin County, California. The college is the American epicenter of learning for students of North Indian classical music, and offers instruction in tabla, as well as the Indian musical instruments sitar and sarod, and singing. It was founded by Ali Akbar Khan, a legendary musician who was considered by many to hold the stature of a contemporary Bach or Beethoven. "Khansahib," as he was called by his students, learned music at the feet of his father, Allauddin Khan, who was also Ravi Shankar's teacher.

It was here in the heady atmosphere of the music college that I came to study with one of the world's greatest living tabla maestros, Pandit Swapan Chaudhuri. Once a week, the other students and I would gather around Swapan with our drums as he demonstrated his exquisite playing and his stunning knowledge of a truly dizzying array of tabla compositions and rhythms. Forbidden from stopping to take notes in the lessons, we were expected to learn to "speak" the tabla rhythms before we attempted to play them on the drums. Every week's lesson was a true leap of faith in my own abilities, but Swapan was a patient and caring teacher who inspired me to dedicate myself fully to learning as much as I could from him.

In one particular lesson, on the day after a truly stellar concert that Ali Akbar Khan and Swapan had given at the Palace of Fine Arts in San Francisco, we were all gathered around as usual. Before launching into the day's lesson, however, some of us in the group were commenting to him about how amazing the concert had been the night before. Being keen students, we had noticed that in one particularly magical moment of the concert, there had been a sudden shift in the rhythm of the music they were performing. They'd been playing along the entire song in an eight-beat rhythm cycle and then, out of nowhere, as the energy of the piece seemed to reach an energetic peak, both Ali Akbar Khan and Swapan suddenly began playing in a radically different, fifteen-beat rhythm cycle. The energy in the room exploded and the audience burst into wild applause for this moment of musical genius.

Although there was a detailed concert program that helpfully listed every *raga* (scale or mode) and *tala* (rhythm) for each of the musical pieces that the legendary duo played that night, this dramatic rhythmic time warp was definitely not listed on the menu. So, naturally, inquiring minds like ours wanted to know: Had they rehearsed this moment in advance, intending all along to include it in the performance? Had the concert promoter simply made a mistake in not listing it in the program?

Swapan paused for a long while, smiling knowingly to himself, seeming to wonder if he should even speak these words out loud. We all sat silently, leaning in to hear what he might say. Finally, he spoke: "There is a presence behind the music, a living presence. She is the one who directs the music and the musicians. We play as She would have us play." His words resonated with soulful depth and sincerity. "No, we never rehearsed that."

I felt so grateful in that moment to be part of the global family of musicians, all brothers and sisters in sharing the tremendous healing art of music. I also felt grateful for the amazing gift of being able learn from true musical legends like Swapan, artists who weren't content to merely attain their own greatness but who were moved to share their gifts with eager students like me. In that moment with Swapan, hearing echoes of my own experiences of musical communion in the world of jazz and now in chanting, I saw that these ecstatic glimpses of oneness, these moments of joyful union, are the living heart and soul of all music and the greatest gift it has to offer.

> Our sages developed music from time immemorial for the mind to take shelter in that pure being which stands apart as one's true self. Real music is not for wealth, not for honors, or not even for the joys of the mind—it is one kind of yoga, a path for realization and salvation to purify your mind and heart and give you longevity.
>
> —ALI AKBAR KHAN

Chapter 7

This Is Your Brain on Bhakti

Practice of japa fills the mind with holy vibrations that neutralize vibrations of material consciousness. There are special incantations used in India, called mantras, which have great vibratory force. Repeating them aloud or mentally—with sincere feeling, intelligent understanding, and intense concentration and determination to persevere until Divine contact is actually felt—produces distinct results; body and mind are charged with power as their vibratory rate is heightened.

—Paramahansa Yogananda

Mantras are truly tools of heart, mind, and energy through which I can cultivate the very best in myself, bringing those qualities forth in my life as it is right now. Mantra practice is a daily opportunity to feel and enjoy an embodied experience of the peace, love, and wisdom within me. To touch that place within every day—even for just a few sweet minutes—changes me because it orients my inner compass toward home, toward wholeness and integration.

It's a testament to the power of this practice that many people can tap into a felt experience of this soulful, integrated quality of mantra right from their very first *Om*. But it's also true that in the beginning stages of mantra practice, it may be tempting to think of this time of self-exploration as somehow separate from our daily lives. We may believe those moments of inner peace and joy exist only when we're sitting on our meditation cushion or that we're somehow just escaping reality for a brief time only to have it return once the practice is over.

However, gradually but inevitably we notice that our practice is bearing fruit in our lives in real and lasting ways. We notice that a welcome sense of distance is opening up between us and our usual habitual emotional reactions, allowing us the grace of choosing different, perhaps healthier, responses in their place. We find that the intentions that brought us to the practice in the first place are now beginning to blossom visibly in our lives in the form of new thoughts, new feelings, and new experiences. We see with our own eyes that mantra and chanting has changed us.

From a scientific perspective, a neurobiologist might say that mantra practice is leveraging the brain's natural ability to reorganize and restructure itself through a phenomenon called neuroplasticity. Up until the late twentieth century, scientists believed that once the miraculous growth and transformation of the brain that takes place from infancy through childhood was complete, that was it. The thinking was that once you've hit early adulthood, what you've got is what you get when it comes to the brain.

However, it's only now in our modern twenty-first century that we're able to peer inside the intricacies of the human brain to begin questioning that earlier assumption that the brain stops growing, and for our purposes, to answer the specific question of why chanting works from a scientific perspective. The advent of cutting-edge imaging technology like fMRI (functional magnetic resonance imaging) is opening a window into previously unseen dimensions of the brain for researchers to explore and understand. The revelations and insights of their discoveries are beginning to provide some real evidence and neuroscience to back up what the yogis and chant lovers around the world have known from experience for aeons: chanting and mantra practice is a powerful tool to transform the way we think, the way we feel, and the way we perceive our world.

Neuroplasticity and Our Changing Brains

The scientific consensus on the potential for new growth and re-wiring in the brain began to dawn in the 1960s with the discovery that the damaged brains of stroke victims were undergoing radical transformations as a way of responding and adapting to the biological damage the stroke had inflicted on them. Essentially, the brains of these stroke victims were taking matters into their own hands, reassigning functions from the stroke-impaired parts of the brain to other healthy and undamaged regions, resulting in the restoration of the stroke victims' brain processes—what is called "functional plasticity."

The online Psychology Dictionary defines this miraculous brain presto-chango as: "Ability of one part of our brain to adapt to losing another part." The American neuroscientist Paul Bach-y-Rita, known as the father of neuroplasticity, explains it like this: "If you are driving from here to Milwaukee, and the main bridge goes out, first you are paralyzed. Then you take old secondary roads through the farmland. Then, as you use these roads more, you find shorter paths to use to get where you want to go, and you start to get there faster." Norman Doidge, MD, the author of *The Brain That Changes Itself*, explains Bach-y-Rita's driving metaphor further, saying, "These 'secondary' neural pathways are 'unmasked' or exposed and strengthened as they are used. The 'unmasking' process is generally thought to be one of the principal ways in which the plastic brain reorganizes itself."[14]

Of the many real-world examples of functional plasticity out there, the story of Daniel Kish is definitely one of the most awe-inspiring. In 2015, the NPR podcast *Invisibilia* featured Daniel's amazing life story in an episode entitled "How to Become Batman." Despite the fact that Daniel had been blind since he was a young child, with fearless determination and the support of his loving mother, he taught himself to "see" using echolocation— making clicking sounds with his mouth and learning about the environment around him from the way those sounds bounced back to him.

Over the course of several years, Daniel developed his bat-like abilities to such a degree that by the time he was a teenage boy—a legally blind teenage boy—he was riding his bike around his neighborhood without assistance. (And yes, he wore a helmet.) As Daniel describes it, even though his actual eyes are completely nonfunctioning, he truly sees the world through his ability to echolocate. Not content to be the world's only real-life Batman, Daniel has since trained many other sight-impaired people to learn how they too can see the world for the first time through echolocation.[15]

Purely as a story about phenomenal human achievement, this is amazing, inspiring stuff. But there's more to this tale and its implications for the miraculous organ between our ears. In 2010 and 2011, researchers conducted fMRI studies to examine the brains of several blind individuals just like Daniel who had also developed the ability to echolocate. What they found was astonishing.

The fMRI studies showed that the visual regions of the brain, previously lying dormant in the absence of optical input from the eyes, were actually doing the auditory work of processing the sound information from the echolocation clicks. In other words, the visual centers in the brain had adapted to the functionality of hearing—normally relegated to a completely different part of the brain—utilizing that information to create a visual perception of sorts.[16]

Structural Plasticity

Fortunately, this ability of the human brain to radically reorganize and optimize itself for our benefit is not at all limited to instances of biological disability, damage, or trauma. There's another far more common form of neuroplasticity, and we're already experiencing it every time we learn and memorize something new. It's called "structural plasticity," the brain's ability to form new neural connections and pathways in response to a new experience or memory. This astounding ability of the brain to reorganize and rewire itself is where we'll dive into our search to understand a bit more about why chanting is so effective and, even more importantly, how we can use this understanding to make our chanting and meditation practice as powerful and transformative as possible.

The foundation for this new understanding of how our brains learn and grow is summarized in the handy little phrase "Neurons that fire together, wire together."[17] Essentially, when we consciously engage in any mental activity repeatedly over a period of time, especially with intensity, the brain gradually imprints those patterns of mental activity on our neural structure.

My introduction to the inspiring science behind neuroplasticity came through the work of Dr. Rick Hanson and his books *Buddha's Brain* and *Hardwiring Happiness*. Dr. Hanson is a neuropsychologist whose life work is to share the surprisingly simple tools and techniques that we can all use to, as he puts it, "use the mind to change the brain to change the mind for the better."[18]

To understand this Escheresque take on brain science, consider how our state of mind and the physical brain that underlies it are inexorably linked, like the software running on our computers. In fact, it's impossible to imagine the entire realm of thought, perception, and feeling existing at all without that inconceivably powerful, three-pound engine of biological hardware under the hood. As Dr. Hanson says, the physical brain is "the master organ of the body and the primary internal source of your well-being, everyday effectiveness, psychological healing, personal growth, creativity and success. Whether you feel angry or at ease, frustrated or fulfilled, lonely or loved depends on your neural networks."[19]

Naturally, then, since a healthy, happy brain makes for a healthy, happy person, we want to do all we can to cultivate the healthiest, happiest brain we possibly can. Fortunately for us, the new science of structural plasticity offers powerful new insights and tools to help us do exactly that.

To encourage us along our journey, let's look at some inspiring examples of how people are expanding and developing their brains through learning and experience.

The Musical Brain

In 2003, two researchers published the findings of an in-depth brain study entitled, "Brain Structures Differ between Musicians and Non-Musicians." For the purposes of their research, they gathered together twenty professional musicians, twenty amateur musicians, and forty non-musicians. To minimize any variables between the test subjects other than their musical abilities, they were all matched for gender, age, and even IQ. All things being equal, one might have expected that these men's brains should look fairly similar.

Instead, what the study revealed was "significant positive correlation between musician status and increase in gray matter volume." The professional musicians were found to have the highest gray matter volume increase (yes!), with enhancements in several regions of the brain including those that control motor, auditory, and visual function. Amateur musicians came in second with moderate gray matter volume enhancement. And the non-musicians, well, they all went home after the study and hopefully signed up for their first singing lessons.[20]

Eight Weeks to a New Brain

Now, to be clear, it won't be necessary for us to learn to play Rachmaninoff on the piano in order to reap the benefits of a supercharged brain. There are simple, everyday things we can all do—and truly enjoy as we're doing them—that have tremendous, lasting impact on our brains' health, well-being, and tendency toward positive, loving, compassionate, peaceful, and joy-filled states of mind.

In 2011, a research team affiliated with Harvard University set out to demonstrate precisely how a simple daily mindfulness meditation practice might positively affect our brains and our well-being. Sixteen subjects participated in the eight-week study, which was directed by Dr. Sara Lazar at Boston General Hospital's Psychiatric Neuroimaging Division. "Although the practice of meditation is associated with a sense of peacefulness and physical relaxation," Lazar says, "practitioners have long claimed that meditation also provides cognitive and psychological benefits that persist throughout the day." By measuring the meditator's brain structure with magnetic resonance imaging before and after the eight-week program, Dr. Lazar hoped to put that claim of meditation's lasting cognitive and psychological benefits to the test.

Participants practiced daily mindfulness meditation as a group and on their own with the support of audio recordings of guided meditations for an average of just twenty-seven minutes a day. The participants also filled out a mindfulness questionnaire at the beginning of the program to assess their own state of well-being and stress levels. After just eight weeks of mindfulness meditation, the researchers compared the before and after images of the meditator's brains. Even the most experienced neuroscientists on the team were astonished by what they saw.

First, the researchers discovered that the part of the brain associated with learning and memory (the hippocampus) had increased in gray matter density. Second, they noticed that other brain structures associated with self-awareness, introspection, and compassion had also noticeably increased. When the participants revisited the mindfulness questionnaire at the end of the study, they reported many significant overall improvements and a reduction in stress. Interestingly, the post-study MR images for the meditators concurred, revealing that their amygdalas (the area of the brain associated with anxiety and stress) had decreased in gray matter density.

As incredible as these results are, they become even more inspiring when we consider the fact that the subjects of the study

were actually new to meditation. All of the changes in the participants' brain structure that were documented by the researchers
were the result of just eight weeks of practice for first-time meditators! Dr. Lazar summed up the program's impressive results:
"This study demonstrates that changes in brain structure may un-
derlie some of these reported improvements and that people are
not just feeling better because they are spending time relaxing."

And this isn't the first time that her research has borne this out.
An earlier study she directed back in 2005 found that experienced
meditators showed noticeable differences in the structure of their
brains—particularly in a thickening of the cerebral cortex—in
areas associated with attention and emotional integration. The
results of the earlier study also suggest that meditation may act
as a preventative against a specific type of age-related decline in
the brain. Britta Hölzel, another member of Dr. Lazar's research
team, sums up the implications of their findings: "It is fascinating
to see the brain's plasticity and that, by practicing meditation, we
can play an active role in changing the brain and can increase our
well-being and quality of life."[21]

You must have a room or a certain hour of the
day . . . a place where you can simply experience
and bring forth what you are, and what you might
be. . . . At first you may find nothing's happening. . . . But if you have a sacred place and use it,
take advantage of it, something will happen.
—JOSEPH CAMPBELL

Bringing It Down Home

Beyond the scientific studies I shared above, many of you have likely already seen, read, and heard just how much science and medicine are now engaged in researching and learning more about the measurable, real-world benefits of meditation and mindfulness. At the same time, even holistic practices like acupuncture and yoga—once deemed "alternative"—are now quite mainstream. It's an exciting time when we see a general increase in conversation and exploration between disciplines—a bridge that can expand our thinking. In the next portion of this chapter we'll continue in this spirit of connection, utilizing the latest insights in neuroscience and finding simple, practical ways to integrate them in order to bring more happiness, love, and well-being into our personal, everyday lives.

To see how an actual neuropsychologist would advise us on cultivating this quality of peace and well-being, what Dr. Rick Hanson calls the "Buddha brain," for ourselves, let's look further into his research for guidance. According to Dr. Hanson, encouraging our brains to become more Buddha-full is as easy as relishing an exquisite sunset, basking in the warm feelings of love for our child or partner, feeling gratitude for someone or something in our lives, or literally any of the other day-to-day momentary glimpses of positive emotions that we each—even on the hard days—can choose to truly notice and allow ourselves to experience more fully.

It sounds simple, and it is, but if we want to parlay these everyday moments of elevated, positive states of mind into real, lasting changes in the brain—whether we find those moments in our daily lives or during our mantra and meditation practice—there are a couple of additional steps that we'll want to take. In his fantastic book *Hardwiring Happiness*, Dr. Hanson teaches a powerful practice that encapsulates his secret recipe for brain change called Taking in the Good. Essentially, there are three steps to the process he's innovated—with a fourth, optional step once we've had some practice with the first three. There's even a handy acronym to help us remember the steps: *HEAL*.

Step 1: Have a positive experience.
Step 2: Enrich and extend that experience.
Step 3: Absorb the energies and qualities of the experience.
Step 4: Link positive and negative material. [22]

Now let's break down each of these steps in depth so that you fully understand the process and put it to good use.

Step One: Having a positive experience. This first step can be as simple as noticing a positive experience that happens naturally through the course of your day, an external event in your life that triggers positive feelings. It can also be an experience that you consciously generate within yourself without any external trigger whatsoever, like choosing to take a moment just to appreciate something you're grateful for. I've even had powerful experiences with this first step while walking through the gate at the airport—just a moment of friendly eye contact between me and the gate agent as I boarded the plane that sparked a feeling of gratitude in me for human connection, for the little ways in which we can support one another and wish each other well, even someone we've never met before.

To be clear, Taking in the Good is about much more than mere positive thinking. The real high-octane fuel for brain change flows when positive thought rises to the level of positive and embodied *feeling*—the more powerful the better.

This brings us to Step Two: Enriching and extending. Turning these everyday moments of positive experience into positive, lasting changes in the brain is, according to neuroscience, simply a matter of time and intensity. (Remember, "Neurons that fire together, wire together.") So, to get those neurons firing and wiring together, we simply allow ourselves to stay with the positive experience for five to ten seconds or more—extending the experience—resisting the natural human tendency to let these moments of goodness pass us by without fully appreciating them. In addition, as we allow ourselves to steep in the experience, we also begin to enrich and amplify it—gently fanning the flames of the positive feelings the experience has sparked in us until they fill our hearts and minds.

We can do this enriching process in one or all of several ways. We can consciously open ourselves to the good feelings we're having, utilizing our breath to intensify and enhance them. (I like to use *ujjayi* breath, the ocean-sounding breath described in the Glossary) to amp up the experience, directing my breath into the place in my body where I'm feeling the positive emotion most strongly.) We can also enrich our experience through thought, contemplating other aspects of the experience and how it will benefit us, the people we love, our community, and the world around us. In any way that's effective for us, we allow ourselves to luxuriate in the healing, positive feelings we've generated in the moment.

Again, to really receive the neurological benefit, it's recommended to stay with the enrichment step for *at least* five to ten seconds. However, the longer we stay with it, the stronger the intensity of the feelings, and the greater the benefit to our brains. It's to our benefit to soak in the healing energies of the elevated feeling state for as long as we feel called to do. Once we feel complete with this step, we'll move on to the next.

Step Three: Absorbing the energies of the experience. In the afterglow of the positive feeling state we've cultivated, we take a moment to consciously draw the energies and qualities of the experience into our bodies and minds. This enhances the benefits of the practice, making it more likely that our positive experience will translate to lasting changes in our neural structure. Again, there are different techniques we can explore to see what works best for us but the idea is to experience the sensation that these positive energies are actually being *absorbed* into us, becoming a part of our mind, heart, and being.

Here are a few ways you might find useful. We can use our breath to inhale the energy into us, drawing it deep inside with each inhalation. We can use the power of visualization to imagine the energy permeating every cell of our being, filling us with the radiant light of its transforming power. We can imagine that the energy is like a warm, gentle rain falling onto our skin and soaking into us. We can place both hands over our heart, feeling the fullness of the healing energy from our experience within us.

Beautifully describing these first three steps of the practice, Dr. Rick Hanson says: "In effect, Taking in the Good is like making a fire. Step 1 lights it, Step 2 adds fuel to keep it going, and Step 3 fills you with its warmth. You can start the third step after clearly ending the second step, but much of the time, the sense of absorbing a positive experience mingles with and overlaps the sense of enriching it. It's like being warmed by a fire even as you add sticks to it."[23]

Once we have the sense that we've really made the practice our own and that we're able to flow comfortably from steps one through three, we might choose to invite the next step into the mix.

Step Four: Linking positive and negative material. While

keeping a strong, embodied sense of the positive experience we've generated in the foreground of our minds, we then also bring to mind a challenging or negative memory somehow related to this new positive experience. For example, if we've cultivated a strong experience of self-love and self-worth, we could then gently bring to mind a memory of a time we doubted ourselves—infusing the old, hurtful memory with the healing energies of our new experience. When we feel complete, we release the challenging memory and return for a few moments to bathing in the positive experience to finish the practice.

It's important in this final part of the practice that the positive experience remains predominate and our primary focus, with the negative material relegated to a secondary position in the background of our awareness. If we find that the challenging material begins to take over, throwing us off our game of positive experience, we can let go of the challenging memory and focus exclusively on the positive feelings again.

This process of linking positive new brain states with negative memory gradually begins to heal the hurt and the emotional charge of the old challenging memory. We've all experienced this firsthand when we find ourselves feeling better after talking over a challenging situation with a caring, supportive friend or counselor. By sifting the healing energies of compassion and love into our hurt places, we find that we naturally start to feel better. And, of course, there's actual neuroscience at work behind this process.

It's in those moments where the brain is reconstituting the memories of our experiences where neuroscience has identified this opening, this opportunity to consciously choose to weave in new, positive feeling and experience into the memory fabric of a challenging one. Over time, leavening the memory of a negative experience with new positive material can gradually dissolve whatever emotional and energetic hold it had on our lives.

Once we've completed the basic process of step four, there's one more little brain-change gem we can utilize to further enhance the healing power of this linking technique. For the next hour or so after we've completed the four steps of the practice, we might choose to revisit the positive experience we generated as often as we'd like. At the same time, we bring to mind the thought of the "neutral trigger," that is, the person, place, or thing that has come to be associated with the challenging experience or feelings.

HEAL with Mantra

The big takeaway from Dr. Hanson's HEAL technique is that I recognize more and more how traditional mantra practice already teaches and embodies the insights that modern science is just discovering. However, the great contribution of brain science in this regard is its ability to accurately pinpoint at least some of the neurological processes that mantra practice is activating. Informing our mantra practice with these new insights into how our brains actually do grow and change can only serve to enhance and empower our practice.

Anytime we give ourselves the gift of mantra practice we're actually already Taking in the Good. However, applying the insights we've just learned to our mantra practice can be a powerful way to deepen our connection and experience with the practice; it also makes it far more likely that the practice will bear fruit for us in the form of personal, emotional, and spiritual growth and transformation. What's more, for many of us there's a lot to be said just for the energizing and confidence-building effects of knowing we have solid, scientifically affirmed ground to stand on as we embark on our mantra journey.

Of course, I'm under no illusions that even our most cutting-edge brain science has completely cracked the code of the infinite power and depth of the human mind, heart, and soul. If anything, discovering that we possess a magically self-transforming brain makes me feel more wonder and awe for the power and intelligence of Life.

Essentially, every single mantra we might choose to chant can become for us an experience of Taking in the Good. Let's repurpose the four steps of HEAL, this time with an eye toward integrating them into our mantra practice.

Step One: Have a positive experience. No matter what variety of mantra practice we happen to be doing—whether we're singing call-and-response at a public kirtan, intoning the ancient sounds of the *Gayatri* mantra from the comfort of home, or silently repeating *Om Namah Shivaya* with our japa mala beads in hand—the moment we begin our mantra practice, we are inviting a powerful experience of the good into our lives in a very proactive way. The beauty of the mantra-based version of this practice is really twofold. First, in bringing this science of brain change into our daily mantra *sadhana* (spiritual practice), we're giving ourselves the gift of consistent, extended, and deep immersion in Taking in the Good rather than waiting for life to present an occasion for us to jump into the practice. Second, having chosen a mantra practice that supports our own personal intentions, we can truly focus and channel the additional benefits of Taking in the Good directly toward those intentions, knowing that we're building a new neural structure in our brains to support our intentions as we do the practice.

Step Two: Enrich and extend that experience. Chanting offers us an abundance of opportunities to enrich and enliven our Taking in the Good practice. To begin with, when our chanting practice includes singing, the healing power of the voice itself can become a vehicle and an expression of the positive energetic and emotional qualities that we seek to cultivate in our practice. As we sing the mantra, we can tune in to the sense that those positive energies and qualities are resonating through our own voice, permeating our entire body.

At the same time, whether singing out loud or repeating a mantra silently, we can call forth the energetic qualities embodied in the archetype of the Deity. For example, if we're chanting a mantra to the God Hanuman, we can cultivate a palpable energetic experience of the qualities of inner strength, courage, and love within ourselves. We can also allow our minds to contemplate the imagery and iconography of the Deity, bringing another facet of inspiration into the practice.

We might also experiment with introducing *mudra* (hand gestures) into our practice to deepen the experience and make it even more powerful by triggering the brain's "embodied cognition" response (the scientific theory that physical experience in the body influences changes in cognition and the brain). Finding a mudra that aligns well with our intentions or that just feels right to us, we can enhance the practice by physically expressing and embodying the energies we're cultivating.

Step Three: Absorb the energies and qualities of the experience. One of my favorite parts of mantra practice is the depth of the sweet, silent space that remains after the practice has finished. This is the perfect time to really draw all that energetic goodness from our practice deeply into ourselves, breathing it in with every breath, our hearts filled with gratitude for the gift of this practice. You might find that the beautiful sound of the tamboura drone (see Chapter 3, "The Drone Zone") is a welcome addition throughout your practice but, most especially, here during these final moments, where the intoxicating vibrations can deeply enhance the sense of bathing in and receiving the positive benefits from our sadhana, or spiritual practice.

We might also choose to do a few minutes of pranayama (yogic breathing) at the end of our practice to balance our energy and further ingrain the new positive qualities and experiences into our system. I like to do four or five rounds of nadi shodhana (alternate nostril breathing) as a way of bringing my practice to a close.

Step Four: Link positive and negative material. Mantra gives us a convenient and reliable way to solidly anchor ourselves in the positive feelings and qualities of our experience as we start to do the work of healing challenging old patterns by weaving in the new, positive material from our practice. Mantra is particularly effective when we're doing the "neutral trigger" technique and we want to call forth the feeling-tone of our positive experience again several times during the hour or so after our initial practice. Simply beginning to repeat the same mantra again, either silently or out loud, will automatically rekindle the energy of our positive experience within us. We can also enhance this part of the practice by reconnecting with a mental image of the Deity whose mantra we're chanting, further deepening our connection with the positive feeling state while we shine that healing, transformative energy onto the background mental image of the neutral trigger. Once we've done this several times over the course of an hour or so and we feel complete, we release the image of the neutral trigger and simply abide in the sweet energy of the positive experience we've created through the practice.

Nothing New Under the Sun

For aeons, yogis, sages, and saints have touted the practice of mantra and meditation as a means to inner peace, happiness, love, and wisdom. Within their words and teachings on the practice of mantra, one theme is ever-present: mantra practice must be done with "sincere feeling . . . intense concentration . . . until Divine contact is actually felt," as Yogananda said in the quote at the beginning of this chapter.[24] The quality of mantra practice that these wise beings described is not merely rote repetition of some mystic incantation. The practice they describe is, instead, an occasion for a deeply felt, powerful, and embodied experience within the mind, heart, and body of the chanter.

It's no coincidence, then, that this experiential, embodied, feeling-based quality of the practice is precisely what neuroscience tells us can bring about a complete reorganizing and upgrading of our neural networks, gradually building the brain structure to support and express greater happiness, joy, and fulfillment in our lives.

As the neuropsychologist Dr. Hanson says, by putting these insights into action through your daily practice you will "turn everyday good experiences into good neural structure. Putting it more technically: You will *activate* mental states and then *install* them as neural traits."[25]

In the next chapter, we'll explore a variety of different modes and styles of this powerful practice, each with its own unique qualities and energetic offerings. In our journey through the various modes of chanting practice, perhaps we'll discover some that are new to us, and learn more about the ones we're already familiar with, inspiring and enlivening our experience of the yoga of chanting.

Chapter 8

The Three Modes of Mantra Practice

One way or another, we all have to find what best fosters the flowering of our humanity in this contemporary life, and dedicate ourselves to that.

—Joseph Campbell

In the yoga of chanting, there is such a bountiful variety of mantras out there for us to explore and experience. That bounty is so great that even though I've been deeply immersed in mantra practice of all kinds for more than twenty years, I still regularly come across mantras that I've never even seen before, let alone actually practiced myself. During the process of writing this book, for example, when I felt called to invite the flowing, creative energies of Saraswati—the Hindu Goddess of music, arts, and wisdom—into my life in a more powerful way, I came across the *Maha Vidya* ("Queen of Knowledge") mantra that you'll see in the Shakti chapter in the Songbook for the Soul. Now, that Saraswati mantra didn't just magically appear out of the ethers; it had been there all along, waiting patiently on page 173 of Thomas Ashley-Farrand's *Healing Mantras* book. Yet, it wasn't until I had arrived at a place in my life when I truly needed the energetic support of this mantra, until I was really ready for it, that I actually found it and embraced it as a practice.

That's the way it works: when we're ready, when we need it, the right mantra appears. It's almost as though the energy of the mantra finds us. Although I'm not quite sure whether it's us attracting the energy of the mantra, or the energy of the mantra attracting us. Either way, when the time is right, the energy of our own unique being aligns with the energy of a particular mantra and we discover the perfect practice to serve our highest intention.

With the overflowing abundance of potential mantras out there for us to explore, it may be clarifying to begin to see that the yoga of chanting actually has just a few basic categories of practice, not unlike the way in which the myriad postures of yoga asanas are helpfully grouped into standing poses, seated poses, twists, inversions, back bends, and so on.

Any yoga teacher can tell you that each of these groupings of yoga postures has its own unique array of qualities and benefits based on the particular way the body is moved and positioned in the asanas of that category. Back bends, for instance, open the heart, shoulders, and chest and are said to offer a natural lift from depression. Inversions improve mental function by increasing blood to the brain, enhance the immune system, build upper-body strength, and literally offer us a new perspective on the world. Mindful of the unique attributes of these different categories of physical postures, a good yoga teacher will weave them all together into a well-rounded, balanced, and effective sequence.

In the same way, by becoming familiar with the qualities and benefits of these basic categories within the yoga of chanting we can weave together an inspiring variety of mantra practices to enrich and enhance our lives. Some of the practices in the yoga of chanting will find us joining our voices with others in a group kirtan, while other practices might find us singing in solitude with the sweet tones of the harmonium or tamboura drone as our only companion. Certain practices will find us enjoying the subtle yet powerful vibrations of the mantra reverberating within our own hearts and minds, with no outward vocalizing of the sound at all. Still other practices will find us expressing the energy of the mantra through the unique process of writing it out on the page or on an image of a Deity. And then, even in the midst of our daily lives, we might find ourselves simply breathing in the sounds of the mantra vibrating within us, allowing the uplifting and healing energy of our practice to carry us through our day.

Now, to be clear, it's possible to chant the very same mantra in many of these different modes of practice. The mantra *Om Namah Shivaya*, for example, could easily be chanted in all of the various modes of practice I just listed above, and each style of chanting would bring out a different nuance of the mantra's energies. Becoming familiar with these various styles and categories of chanting will support us in getting the most out of our chosen mantra and our practice in general.

Group Chanting:
Answering the Call of Kirtan

Within the body there is played
Music unending, though without stringed instruments.
That music of the Word pervades the entire creation.
Who listens to it is freed from all illusion.

—KABIR

We'll begin our journey through the categories in the yoga of chanting with the form of mantra practice that is certainly the most widely known, not only here in America but around the world. Group chanting includes the popular practice of kirtan: call-and-response singing of the mantra with the dynamic accompaniment of musical instruments. Kirtan is a powerful, high-energy form of chanting fueled by the undeniable goodness that happens when a room full of people join their voices as one. We've already seen from a scientific perspective just how powerful group singing is in its ability to enhance our physical and emotional well-being, fill our brains with warm, yummy endorphins and oxytocin, and inspire feelings of joyful connection and bonding. When we add to that already potent mix the ancient and powerful energies of mantra, it's easy to see why the kirtan experience has become a worldwide phenomenon.

The next time you happen to find yourself singing *Om Namah Shivaya* at the top of your lungs at a kirtan, think about the fact that your voice is not only joining with all of the other singers in that room but, in reality, with a vast choir of voices that's been growing since the birth of kirtan way back in the seventh century. Kirtan and chanting first became popular with the emergence of the Bhakti movement nearly 1,300 years ago in India, beginning first in the south in what is now Tamil Nadu and gradually migrating north.

The word *bhakti* is often translated as "devotion," but a closer examination of the roots of the word reveals a more nuanced meaning. The Sanskrit word *bhakti* finds its root in the word *bhaj*, which means "to be connected with" or "to belong to." On one level, the Bhakti Yoga practice of kirtan allows us to come together in harmony to share the experience of being connected and belonging to our community. Along this line, many scholars have noted

Bhakti's emphasis on equality, social justice, and religious harmony, welcoming all and everyone into the community of yoga. Taking this idea of connection to an even deeper level, however, the practices of Bhakti Yoga seek to give us a direct experience of our connection with source, Spirit, or the Divine. Rather than espousing the need for some sanctified intermediary—whether priest, church, or ritual—Bhakti Yoga teaches a path of direct personal and devotional relationship with the Divine. The practices of Bhakti Yoga, including chanting as a central component, are intended to cultivate direct experiences of that Divine presence.

Each and every one of the modes of mantra practice that we'll explore in this chapter arises from this path of the heart known as Bhakti Yoga. However, as we'll see, each has its own unique flavor. Here in the realm of kirtan, for example, the practice is celebratory and community-oriented. Musicians are essential to making the magic of kirtan happen, even if it's just one guy banging on a drum or clanging some finger cymbals while someone else leads the chanting. Although that simple instrumentation can work perfectly well and it's probably quite similar to how the kirtan *wallahs* (leaders) used to roll back in the old days, the musical instrumentation of a contemporary kirtan is far more eclectic. Whether we hear slide guitar, drum kit, cello, or synthesizer joining into the musical offering, however, the devotional quality of a kirtan now should be exactly the same as it's always been. We should feel transported by a heart-wave of energy and love flowing through the music and the mantras.

Soaring with the Birds: Meditation Mantras

Although the call-and-response style of kirtan is the most widely known form of group chanting, there are many other mantra practices we can experience in this category as well. For instance, the power of group singing can be used to amplify and enhance the experience of chanting longer meditation mantras such as the *Gayatri, Mahamrityunjaya, Lokah Samasthah,* and others. Then there's the beautiful, slow meditation style of chanting a simple mantra such as *Om Shri Durgayai Namah* or *Om Namah Shivaya* that is tremendously powerful when chanted in a group (see Chapters 16 and 17). This style of chanting is deep and introspective, with a rhythm that is organic and flowing so that each word of the mantra lasts for one entire exhale rather than for a certain number of beats at a certain tempo. Not surprisingly, this particular slow style of chanting can easily align with the powerful six-breaths-per-minute rhythm we learned about in Part One of the book.

To sing this style of chanting in a group is quite different from the pulsing, dynamic rhythms of kirtan. In this slow, meditative style, if the voices of the group are to come together as one—like a flock of birds, or a school of fish moving in unison—then everyone in the group must listen attentively to the people next to them and match their voice as best they can. It's a beautiful thing to hear how a big group of people who sound very much like a room full of separate individuals in the beginning of a chant will—in a matter of minutes—begin to sing with one unified voice, as if they've become a single being. With their voices, their breathing, and—as we learned from the scientific research—even their brainwaves and their heart rhythms all syncing up to one another, in many ways they really have.

Group chanting holds a uniquely enticing and engaging place among these basic categories of mantra practice. For many people, in fact, it's the only mode of practice they've ever encountered. In the next stop of our journey through the various categories of the yoga of chanting we'll explore a form of mantra practice that is much less familiar even though it's literally right at our fingertips.

Japa Mantra

> If you know who it is that is doing japa you will know what japa is. If you search and try to find out who it is that is doing japa, that japa itself becomes the Self.
>
> —RAMANA MAHARSHI

The second mode of mantra practice is one of the most powerful forms that requires no musical accompaniment at all, one that we can enjoy anytime we feel inspired to, rather than at the fixed time of a public kirtan event, and one that allows us to dive deeply and one-pointedly into the mantra that we've chosen to support us in our highest intentions. *Japa* is a Sanskrit word that means "to repeat or to chant in a low voice or a whisper." In this form of chanting practice, we steep ourselves in the energy and vibration of our mantra through mindful and heartfelt repetition. As we'll see, there are a few different tools available to support us in this empowering and healing form of mantra practice.

Bliss at Your Fingertips: Japa Mala Practice

A mala is a necklace of prayer beads, a rosary that serves as a worthy ally in the practice of japa. As each of the 108 beads of the mala passes between our fingers, we repeat the sound of our mantra. The mala is traditionally held in the right hand, between the thumb and the middle finger. Although, if you're left-handed and you feel more comfortable switching it up, I'm sure Lord Shiva won't mind. You'll notice that malas have one bead that's usually a bit larger or made from a different material than the rest. This unique bead is the *meru* bead and it's a handy way to know when you've reached the end of your 108-mantra repetitions, should you be going more than one time around the mala. Traditionally, once you reach the meru bead, you turn the mala around in your hand and begin your next round using the bead you just finished on. I like to hold my mala in front of my heart to bring forth as much feeling into the practice as possible, using ujjayi breath to amplify the inner resonance of the mantra.

You might also enhance your japa practice by choosing a mala made from a certain gemstone, crystal, or wood that feels good for you. You can find malas made from your birthstone, from gemstones said to activate a certain chakra or to possess particular healing energies, or from traditional materials such as *rudraksha* seeds, which are said to clear negative karmic energies. The best kind of mala to choose, however, is the one that supports you in feeling inspired and energized when you practice. In the back of this book in the Recommended Resources Guide you'll find details on where you can get beautiful malas of all varieties.

Once we've got our mala in hand and we're ready to begin our japa practice with the mantra of our choice, we simply begin repeating the sounds of the mantra with as much attention, focus, and feeling as we can muster. In the beginning, that repetition may be spoken audibly, especially as we're getting familiar with the sound of a new mantra. However, as we progress with japa practice, we find that the vibrations of the mantra gradually descend deeper and deeper into us. Soon, the audible, external practice naturally falls away as we become attuned to the inner resonance of the mantra. The mind and heart become one-pointed on the vibrations of the chant reverberating within us, as we steep ourselves in the energetic qualities of the mantra.

A japa practice usually involves doing a certain number of "rounds" (once around the mala, or 108 repetitions) on a daily basis. If we've chosen to dedicate at least ten to fifteen minutes a day to this style of mantra practice, we'll find that we can get through five rounds or so of a shorter mantra like *Om Gam Ganapatayai Namah*, while a longer mantra like the *Gayatri* would easily fill up an entire fifteen-minute japa session (and then some) with just one round of 108. Creating a daily mantra practice, or sadhana, for yourself is as simple as aligning three things: the amount of time you'd like to dedicate to your practice every day, the mantra that you feel called to use, and how many rounds of that mantra you can do in the time you've set aside for your practice.

To really amplify the benefits and the energies generated from your japa practice, you might feel inspired to embrace another beautiful yogic tradition called an *anusthan*. When you do an anusthan, you commit to doing your mantra practice a certain number of times (whether it's one round or ten rounds) for a set number of days (often forty) without missing a day of practice. This dedicated period of unbroken practice is an effective means of establishing a new energetic pattern in yourself and signaling your highest intentions to the Universe in a focused and powerful way. And at the end of the book, I offer this practice with instructions for you to create your own intentional anusthan experience. It's an incredible practice that has given me amazing results and benefits—it's a way to truly focus and empower your mantra with purpose.

Whether you're doing japa as part of a special, dedicated 40-

day anusthan or simply as an ongoing daily practice, you are utilizing the powerful, transformational tool of mantra to cultivate happiness, peace, well-being, wisdom, love, and all the highest human virtues in a direct, experiential way that will undoubtedly radiate into your life in noticeable, often amazing ways. When we enliven our japa mantra by infusing it with the feeling-tone of our intentions, the benefits and depth of experience from the practice increase exponentially. Rather than simply reciting our mantra in a mechanical way, it should become like our favorite song playing in our heart.

Skywriting in the Mind: Likhita Japa Practice

The specialty of mantra writing is that our whole consciousness is involved in it. Action, thought, and emotion become one. In this way, all the three powers—the power of action, the power of thought and the power of emotion—are unified. While chanting, the mind may wander here and there, but while writing, it cannot go anywhere and hence one can do it with full concentration.

—SHRI RAMESH BHAI OJHA

While mantra practice can take many different forms, there is one particular kind of mantra practice that is truly unique. Whereas all of the other mantra practices rely upon some type of recitation—whether sung, spoken, or heard internally with the inner ears—*likhita japa* expands on the practice by adding a visual component: the writing out of the mantras by hand.

In likhita japa, one writes the mantra or Divine Name repeatedly while contemplating the qualities, energies, and attributes of the mantra or the Deity whose name is being written. This fusion of contemplation and written mantra practice engages a dynamic conversation between the mind and the heart, between symbol and meaning, and, in fact, between the left and right hemispheres of the brain.

There is something uniquely powerful about linking the energy of mantra with the everyday act of writing. We're so used to employing the written word as an expression of conceptual, rational thought. But in the realm of the likhita practice, the boundaries of the written word are expanded to embody and express the archetypal and mythic energy of mantra. This brings a certain transcendent quality to the likhita practice, as we connect to the Infinite through the finite means of the written word.

For many people, myself included, this is one of the most accessible and engaging of all of the mantra practices. I like to think of likhita japa as a kind of "skywriting in the mind." Thoughts follow where the ink flows and the mind is entrained by the rhythm of the mantra as you write again and again. I find that this practice has an almost magical power to calm and focus an active mind, bringing the whole being into a state of contemplative ease in a short period of time.

As with all of the other styles of practice that we've explored, any mantra that you feel connected to, that feels meaningful for you, is a great choice for likhita japa practice. That said, it's usually a good idea in the beginning to work with mantras that are on the shorter side (rather than, say, the twenty-four-syllable *Gayatri* mantra). A mantra that fits easily within one written line is a good place to start. You may also find it empowering to get yourself a special pen and notebook that's dedicated solely to your likhita japa. This can enhance the power of your practice by allowing the subtle energies of the written mantras to build up over time. Keep your special pen and notebook in your altar or, alternatively, in a nightstand near your bed. This way, you can absorb the good energies you've generated while you sleep.

If you'd like, you can choose to write your mantra a certain number of times a day. As we've seen with other forms of mantra practice, particular numbers are said to hold special, auspicious power: 9, 27, 54, and 108 are the ones most often recommended. Or, if you'd rather, you can simply write without keeping count and just enjoy the practice for as long as you like.

As you write your mantra, allow your mind to dwell on the energetic qualities of the mantra or Deity. Listen with your inner ears and attune yourself to the vibrations of the mantra as it resonates within you. Imagine that you're writing these sacred syllables within your own heart and mind, not merely on paper. Once your writing practice is complete, allow yourself time to sit in meditation for at least five minutes. Soak in the energies of the practice. You may wish to do a few rounds of pranayama (yogic breathing) to help circulate the energy; nadhi shodhana (alternate nostril breathing) is a great choice.

As with any of the other forms of mantra sadhanas we've explored, using a tamboura drone can enhance the practice of likhita japa. And since there's no singing to be done in this practice, we're free to choose any key for our drone that appeals to us, regardless of how it might relate to our vocal sweet spot. For example, I really enjoy using a drone in the key of B for this kind of practice, although this key would be a bit low for me vocally if I were singing. Experiment, and see what key feels best to you. You may also find further inspiration in the "Drone Zone" chapter. In particular, have a look at the chart that correlates the various musical keys with the chakra system and see if any of the energetic qualities of the chakras resonate with your intentions for doing your likhita practice.

Sacred Shapes

Another powerful way to do likhita practice is to abandon the linear style of writing altogether. The mantra is written instead upon an inspiring image that gives expression to the Deity, archetype, or energy of the mantra. Many people find this more artistic expression of the practice to be particularly heart-opening and engaging. Here's how you can do it:

1. First, look for an image that deeply inspires you and print it out. Simple illustrations and line drawings work very well for this since they offer more open space. Also, it goes without saying that the bigger the image, the more room to write. An image that fills an 8.5-by-11-inch sheet of paper is a perfect size.

2. Now that you have your image and you're ready to begin your practice, take a few deep breaths. Exhale slowly, releasing any tension in the body. As you take up your pen to begin writing, simply write your mantra wherever and however your heart and mind feel called to write it. There are no rules.

3. Allow your eyes to take in the quality of the sacred image and to allow that quality to inspire your writing and inner chanting of the mantra. Flow with the practice and let it lead you into deeper and deeper states of immersion.

4. When you feel complete with your practice, take a few minutes to sit in meditation. You may want to begin by

gazing at the image, now enlivened through your mantra practice. Breathe in the energy you feel radiating from the image. Allow the sound of your mantra to continue resonating within you with each inhale and exhale. Explore ujjayi breath to help strengthen the vibration of the inner mantra.

Every Breath You Take: Ajapa Japa

Our last stop in the category of japa mantra is the subtlest, deepest practice of all, one that usually only arises naturally once we've immersed ourselves for some time in another, more active form of practice. *Ajapa japa* is the internal practice of merging the sound of the mantra with our breath; essentially, breathing our mantra in and out. We can engage in the practice intentionally, calling forth the healing vibrations of our mantra with our breath throughout the day. In the highest expression of this practice, however, ajapa arises spontaneously, automatically, without any additional effort on our part. Once our mantra has become so deeply ingrained in us, its sacred rhythm goes on all the time like a heartbeat.

One familiar version of the ajapa breath practice is the famous *So'ham* mantra, which is pronounced as "so hum." The mantra is really an affirmation of our true spiritual nature with every breath. This affirmation is reflected both in the literal meaning of the Sanksrit ("I am He" or "I am That") as well as in the fact that the sounds of the mantra are very much like those we make naturally when we breathe, with "So" on the inhale and "hum" on the exhale.

Try it once for yourself right now, noticing that your inhale naturally has an "oh" sound quality as you open yourself to receive oxygen, while your exhale naturally has a "hum" quality as the spent air is released. The *So'ham* breath practice simply enhances this naturally occurring mantra of our own breath, inviting conscious awareness of our Divine nature with every inhale and every exhale.

Since the sound of our own breathing aligns so perfectly with this *So'ham* style of breath practice, serving as an innate reminder to return again and again to our mantra, we might be inspired to use this same style with a different mantra to create a breath practice that feels more closely connected to our own intentions. If we're already doing a Lakshmi mantra as part of our japa mala practice, for instance, we could easily create a *So'ham*-style breath practice by using a *bija* mantra for Lakshmi. The word *bija* means "seed" and it refers to a highly condensed and powerful form of mantra that is said to embody all the energetic qualities of the Deity or Divine archetype within its primal sound vibrations. The mantra *Om*, for example, is a well-known bija mantra. Creating our own *So'ham*-style practice, we can simply breathe in the sound *Om* and then breathe out the bija of whichever Divine archetype we've chosen.

Here's a list of bija mantras to get you started:

Ganesh—*Gam*
Lakshmi—*Shreem*
Durga—*Dum*
Saraswati—*Aim*
Hanuman—*Hum*
Shiva—*Haum*
Krishna—*Kleem*

This style of breath mantra is a powerful way to stay connected with the energies of our practice throughout the day. You'll also notice that these bija mantras are often included in the longer sad-hana mantras that you'll be using for japa practice. For instance, you might be using the Ganesh mantra *Om Gam Ganapatayai Namah* for your daily japa practice. Then, to connect with the auspicious, obstacle-dissolving energies of Ganesh throughout your day, you could simply inhale *Om* and exhale *Gam*. This is a beautiful way to keep the uplifting and healing energy of mantra flowing throughout your day.

Text Chants: Chalisas, Stotrams, and Mantra Hymns

In the category of text chants, we find a very particular kind of mantra practice, one that serves a dual role of imparting yogic wisdom while also offering a deeply immersive, extended chanting experience. Chants like the *Hanuman Chalisa, Devi Suktam, Nirvanashatkam*—all contained in this book—plus countless others, belong to a unique breed of chanting practice that can be thought of as mantra songs or hymns.

The first feature that makes the chants in this category unique is their length. Whereas each of the chanting styles that we've explored so far typically utilizes mantras from one (like *Om*) to, at most, thirty-three syllables in length (like the *Mahamrityunjaya*), the text chants range in length anywhere from 6 to 108 complete verses each, with each verse containing around twenty-four syllables or more. While each and every one of those verses is truly a mantra in and of itself, offering the uplifting and healing experience that comes from chanting sacred sound vibrations, the verses of a text chant also serve another, different yet complementary purpose: each verse of a text chant is a little gem of yogic wisdom, there for our minds to contemplate as we immerse ourselves in the healing sound current of the mantras.

In every verse of the *Hanuman Chalisa*, for instance, we learn the mythology and stories of Hanuman as if we were reading them from the *Ramayana*, the Indian epic scripture that details the life of Rama, seen in the Hindu tradition as a Divine being like Christ. Or in the *Nirvanashatkam*, where the transcendent wisdom of Shiva conveyed in each verse reminds us of our true Self, our minds lifted into the exalted heights of spiritual vision. In this way, the text chants bring an element of Jnana Yoga (the yoga of wisdom) into our chanting practice, initiating a dynamic, inspiring dance between the mind and the heart—between wisdom and love.

In many ways, the text chants offer one of the most immersive and engaging chanting experiences of all, simply because there is a constant stream of ever-changing mantra and meaning flowing through the practice. One feels carried along by the powerful current of sound vibration and wisdom coursing through the chant. As the chant becomes more and more familiar, this dance between the heart and the mind becomes a dynamic form of meditation as you flow from verse to verse.

Strategies for Learning the Text Chants

In an advanced practice like the *Hanuman Chalisa* or any of the other text chants, the sheer volume of unfamiliar words and sounds can be daunting at first. Take heart in the realization that millions of people have learned the very chant that you are now aspiring to learn yourself. Many of them, in fact, are able to recite such epic mantra masterpieces by heart, unaided by any written text at all.

While the memorization of a fairly long and complicated chant such as the *Chalisa* may seem nearly impossible at first glance, there are a few tried-and-true methods we can utilize in order to become text chant aficionados. Be patient with yourself. Through regular practice and a few inside tips, you'll be rocking the text chants in no time.

Mantra Osmosis

One of the most effective ways that I know of to become familiar with a new mantra—whether short, medium, or supersized—is to simply surround ourselves with the sounds of the chant we're seeking to learn. On the old cherrywood credenza in my living room there's an ancient first-generation iPod that I reserve for one purpose and one purpose only: the playing of mantras. I like to refer to my little digital mantra jukebox as "the God Pod."

When I decided to memorize the *Hanuman Chalisa*, I put it on constant repeat so that it was playing in the background day and night. Then, as I went about my daily routine, my attention would naturally drift back to the sound of the chant from time to time. I'd sing along out loud or in my mind with whatever verse happened to be rolling by, then I'd go back to whatever I was doing, allowing the chant to serve as the soundtrack to my day. At least once a day, I'd also actually sit down and chant the entire *Chalisa* with the support of my chant book, looking away from the pages whenever I could recall the words from memory. Over time, through a kind of mantra osmosis, every verse of the *Hanuman Chalisa* gradually encoded itself into my mind and heart so that I can easily recite all forty-some verses from memory. I like to think that I've installed it as a kind of spiritual software into the operating system of my being.

Although the concept of memorizing a long chant like the *Chalisa* may seem impossible at first, it's easier than we might think because the words and sounds of the text chants naturally form a kind of musical link with one another, allowing the entire chant to become familiar and ingrained into us. In my experience, when I reach the end of one memorized verse, that's when the next verse begins to emerge in my mind. It's a little pre-echo of the sounds to come. It's this living link—one verse connected to the next verse connected to the next verse—that strings the entire thing together. It's kind of like the hand bone is connected to the wrist bone, the wrist bone is connected to the arm bone, the arm bone is connected to the shoulder bone, and on and on until you have an entire body. Over time, the verses of the *Chalisa* or any of these extended mantra compositions link together to form a complete whole.

Phone a Friend

There's also no need to go it alone in your journey of learning a text chant. You'll find that there are like-minded folks in your chanting community who, just like you, have always wanted to learn the *Hanuman Chalisa* or another of the text chants but just couldn't quite bring themselves to jump into the practice on their own. In learning the text chants, just as in swimming, the buddy system is always a great idea. Gathering together a little group of two or more people will provide support, encouragement, and connection to sustain you as you get more and more familiar with the practice.

When I first learned the text chants, I was nurtured and supported by the ashram community, where I had the benefit of learning from those who were already deeply familiar with the mantras. If you seek them out, you can certainly find spiritual communities out there where you'll be able join an ongoing text chant practice of one kind or another. However, you can also seek support in your text chant journey by simply singing along with your favorite recording of the chant you'd like to learn. Among the audio links included with this book, you'll find my renditions of the *Hanuman Chalisa, Devi Suktam,* and the *Nirvanashatkam* if you'd like sing along with me as part of your practice.

In the Songbook for the Soul section of the book, you'll find a wide variety of mantras and chants that you can explore in the various styles of chanting that we've discussed in this chapter. There are mantras there of all shapes and sizes, embodying a radiant array of energetic qualities and Divine archetypes. May your chanting practice be filled with love, joy, and wisdom!

Chapter 9

The Three Sounds of *Om*

Om is the one search of all the sciences.

Om is the one goal of all souls.

Om is the One Truth which is worshipped in diverse ways.

Om brings equilibrium. *Om* brings wisdom.

Om is the root. *Om* is the support.

Om pervades all. *Om* sustains all.

Om brings peace, bliss, and power.

Om dissolves the ego, desires, and doubt.

Om is the abode of the soul.

Om is the language of God.

Om is expressed by God.

Om is God.

—Sadguru Sant Keshavadas

If you've spent any time at all in the kirtan community, delved into the *Yoga Sutras of Patanjali* as part of your yoga teacher training, or explored the *Upanishads* or another of the ancient scriptures of India—perhaps in a college philosophy class, as I did—you're probably already well aware of the ever-present *Om* that signals the beginning of most mantras, scriptural verses, meditations, and, for that matter, quite a lot of yoga classes, too. But what exactly is *Om*, really, and why are the yogis so darn fond of it?

We would do well to check in with the authority of the Indian scriptures, where we'll find verse after verse extolling the awesomeness of *Om*. The *Upanishads*, for example, are a deeply inspiring collection of over one hundred spiritual texts, the oldest of which date back to somewhere between 800 and 400 BC. The Sanskrit scholar Juan Mascaró describes them beautifully by saying, "The spirit of the *Upanishads* can be compared with that of the New Testament summed up in the words 'I and my Father are one' and 'The kingdom of God is within you.'"[26]

In our search for "the real *Om*," let's zero in for a moment on just one of the *Upanishads*, the *Mandukya*. Although it's the shortest of all the *Upanishads*, the *Mandukya* is revered as one of the most powerful, and each of its twelve verses offers deep insights about the meaning and the practice of *Om*. To get a taste for the flavor of the yogic wisdom the *Mandukya* has to offer, here are the opening verses:

> *Om*. This eternal Word is all: What was, what is and
> what shall be, and what beyond is in eternity. All is *Om*.
> The first sound A is the first state of waking
> consciousness, common to all men.
> The second sound U is the second state
> of dreaming consciousness.
> The third sound M is the third state
> of sleeping consciousness.
> The word *Om* as one sound is the fourth state of supreme
> consciousness (Turiya). It is beyond the senses and
> is the end of evolution. It is non-duality and love.

He goes with his self to the supreme Self
who knows this, who knows this.
She goes with her self to the supreme Self
who knows this, who knows this.[27]

As we can see from this *Upanishad, Om* is not merely a word but, rather, is meant as a kind of shorthand symbol to signify an *experience* of deep, cosmic union with our higher Self beyond all the triune expressions of existence:

+ **Three states of consciousness:**
  Waking, Dreaming, and Deep Sleep
+ **Three cosmic processes:**
  Creation, Preservation, and Destruction
+ **Three planes of existence:**
  Gross/Physical, Subtle/Mental, and Causal/Karmic
+ **Three levels of mind:**
  Conscious, Unconscious, and Subconscious

Somehow, the sound of *Om*—within its single, solitary syllable—conveys the experience of our true Self beyond all of these existential trinities. But in the same way that we won't get our feet wet in the Pacific Ocean by merely looking at a map of Natural Bridges Beach here in Santa Cruz, California, we won't have this transcendent experience of non-duality and love that *Om* represents merely by reading about it in a scripture. If we want to get our feet wet, we'll have to actually go to the ocean.

This chapter is meant to be a sort of experiential guided tour of the ocean of *Om*. We've heard what the yogis and the scriptures have to say about "the first sound," but unless we can find a way to experience it for ourselves, it's like thinking you're going to get wet from that map of the beach. So, we'll dive deeply into the sound of *Om* in a way that will allow us to experience the subtler nuances of its vibrations. We'll explore the three sounds of *Om*—"A," "U," and "M,"—and by tuning in to these individual primal sound components, we'll truly experience the meaning of the mantra in a way that will allow us to come up with our own definition and understanding of *Om*. Then, with a little luck, if we're paying close attention, we might experience the deeper, inner *Om*. The one that's shining as the blissful, living vibration of consciousness within us all.

Tuning In to the Inner *Om*

As we move through the experience of the three sounds of *Om*, we might find ourselves spontaneously drawn deeper within ourselves to the healing vibrations that our practice has generated. It's really a kind of subtle call-and-response, as if an internal kirtan is unfolding within our own bodies: we sing out the mantra *Om*, and then, if we listen closely, we can hear the subtle but powerful reverberations of our inner *Om* responding back like an echo. This deep, inner listening is one of the great fruits of chanting practice. When the inner mantra begins to shine, our awareness naturally flows toward this vibrational experience within us and we find ourselves drawn into meditation on the *Om* inside.

The truth is, the inner *Om* was inherently there within us even before we started singing. It's just that we become aware of it by attuning ourselves to it through our voices.

I can offer a simple musical analogy for this experience. Whenever I play music in my travels around the world, I typically have two instruments by my side: a guitar and a harmonium. If I were to play a certain note on the harmonium—an E, for example—and if I were to play it nice and loud, there would be an audible response from the guitar. If you were to place your ear up close, you'd hear the E strings of the guitar quietly vibrating. It's not that I have telekinetic powers or anything, it's just physics.

You see, the guitar happens to have two strings that are tuned to that same E note that I played on the harmonium. The correlation in the vibrational frequency between the metal reeds of the harmonium and the steel strings of the guitar sets those strings in motion and they begin to vibrate at their own, innate "E-ness." If you've ever been at a concert where the sweet sound of music is suddenly interrupted by the squeal of feedback, you've experienced this phenomenon of vibrational resonance taken to its unpleasant extreme.

So it is with us. We sing *Om* out loud and, lo and behold, our own innate, internal *Om* begins to resonate within us. This is how the mantra *Om* really came into being in the first place: meditating yogis experienced the bliss of the inner *Om* and found that, if they replicated the sound of *Om* by singing it—matching the vibrational frequency in a way, like the harmonium and the guitar—the inner *Om* would naturally begin to shine forth in response. This is known as the *anahata nada*, "the unstruck sound," because it's always there, vibrating as the blissful sound current of consciousness itself. This is what we're calling the inner *Om*.

Now, the inner *Om* may not show up for us right away. In fact, we may have to keep up our singing *Om* practice for a while before we notice anything at all. But eventually and inevitably the subtle vibrations of the inner *Om* will stir within us. And when they do, what you'll notice is that the inner *Om* is not so much *heard* as it is *felt*. It's a vibrational quality or experience within us that invites us to turn deeper inside, to come home to ourselves. Have you ever noticed that the word *home* has *Om* hidden within it? It's as if the very vibrations of those sounds embody the qualities of refuge, belonging, safety, and arrival. In the course of chanting the three sounds of *Om*, we'll experience those energetic qualities for ourselves.

The thing to remember is that no matter which mantra we might be chanting—from *Om* to the *Gayatri* to the *Hanuman Chalisa*—each and every mantra that we can sing with our mouths can and should also be experienced within us in its subtle vibrational form. To get in the habit of listening for this internal vibration really is an essential part of mantra practice. As you're chanting, keep your inner ear open to the subtle vibrations that begin to arise during your practice. When they do, allow your awareness to follow naturally inward, using the breath to fan the flames of the resonance of the mantra within you.

> The knower of the mystery of sound knows
> the mystery of the whole universe.
> —HAZRAT INAYAT KHAN

Alphabetically Speaking

Even though *Om* is often written in the way that you see here with just two letters, when we consult the original Sanskrit script (called *Devanagari*) for this particular mantra, we can clearly see that there are actually three sounds at play in *Om*: There's an "A," a "U," and an "M." So, what gives?

Well-intentioned scholars and lovers of mantra and Sanskrit wanted to share the gift of this sacred language with as many people as possible. Translating the mantras from the original Sanskrit meant that all of us wouldn't be required to learn to read the ancient Devanagari script ourselves in order to access this bounty of yogic wisdom. The challenge arises from the fact that Sanskrit utilizes a completely different alphabet with far more sounds than the English language. If you consider the fact that there are forty-six different letters in the Devanagari alphabet of Sanskrit compared to twenty-six letters in English, you begin to understand how certain nuances of the language might get lost in translation.

To be clear, though, it's not that writing *AUM* as *Om* is wrong. In fact if you say "A-U-M" quickly, it does sound a lot like *Om* and it's probably a bit less confusing to read it in the simplified, two-letter form as well. For our purposes in this in-depth practice, however, we're really going to dive deep into the essence of the mantra and, with that in mind, we'll be using all three sounds of *Om* to explore the subtle nuances of this ancient chant.

The Three Sounds of *Om*

For our chanting practice, you'll want to set yourself up to be seated comfortably in an upright position either on the floor or in a chair. You can choose to experience this practice one of two ways—either singing along with the audio link below or by simply singing on your own with the support of a tamboura drone. If you choose to fly solo with this practice, you can feel free to tune your drone to your own vocal sweet spot, whereas our shared, prerecorded version of the practice is set in the key of C. Once you're sitting comfortably, we'll begin.

The Three Sounds of *Om*: GirishMusic.com/BookAudio

The first sound of Om is "A," which sounds like "Ah":

1. Take a full inhale and sing "A" ("Ah") for the full length of your exhale, trying to sustain the sound for as long as you comfortably can. As you sing, place your awareness at your sacral center at the root of the spine (Muladhara), sensing that the sound of "Ah" is emanating from there.

2. Take another full inhale and sing "A" ("Ah") a second time, placing your awareness again on the root center. Allow the vibrations of the sound to resonate throughout your entire body.

3. Take another full inhale and sing "A" ("Ah") a third time in the same way. Notice if there's a particular energetic quality or color that you experience with the sound.

4. Resting in silence with eyes closed, allow yourself to hear the sound "A" ("Ah") within yourself.

Think about how we use the sound "Ah" in everyday conversation. What are the qualities conveyed in this sound? Here are a few common ones:

I see
Release

Opening
Wonder
Expansion

The second sound of Om is "U," like "Oo" in pool:

1. Take a full inhale and sing "U" ("Oo") for the full
   length of your exhale, trying to sustain the sound for
   as long as you comfortably can. As you sing, place your
   awareness at your heart center in the center of your chest
   (Anahata), sensing that the sound of "Oo" is emanating
   from there.
2. Take another full inhale and sing "U" ("Oo") a second
   time, placing your awareness again on the heart
   center. Allow the vibrations of the sound to resonate
   throughout your entire body.
3. Take another full inhale and sing "U" ("Oo") a third time
   in the same way. Notice if there's a particular energetic
   quality or color that you experience with the sound.
4. Resting in silence with eyes closed, allow yourself to hear
   the sound "U" ("Oo") within yourself.

Think about how we use the sound "Oo" in everyday conversation. What are the qualities conveyed in this sound? Here are a
few common ones:

Delight
Love
Joy
Revelation

The third sound of Om is "M," which sounds like "Mm":

1. Take a full inhale and sing "M" ("Mm") for the full length of your exhale, trying to sustain the sound for as long as you comfortably can. As you sing, place your awareness at your throat and third-eye center in the middle of your forehead, sensing that the sound of "Mm" is emanating from there.

2. Take another full inhale and sing "M" ("Mm") a second time, placing your awareness again on the throat (Vishuddha) and third-eye (Ajna) centers. Allow the vibrations of the sound to resonate throughout your entire body.

3. Take another full inhale and sing "M" ("Mm") a third time in the same way. Notice if there's a particular energetic quality or color that you experience with the sound.

4. Resting in silence with eyes closed, allow yourself to hear the sound "M" ("Mm") within yourself.

Think about how we use the sound "Mm" in everyday conversation. What are the qualities conveyed in this sound? Here are a few common ones:

Savoring an inner sweetness
"Mmm-mmm good"
Connection
I understand

Merging the Three Sounds of *Om*

Now that we've experienced the three sounds of *Om* individually, we'll merge them together into one connected sound:

1. Take a full inhale. Now chant each of the three sounds of *Om*—"A" ("Ah"), "U" ("Oo"), and "M" ("Mm")—over the course of one exhalation. Allow each of the three sounds to take up an equal third of your exhalation so that they are balanced with one another.

2. As you continue to chant the three sounds of *Om* in succession in this way, tune in to the same sense of placement in the body for each of the sounds as before, with "A" at the Muladhara (root center), "U" at the Anahata (heart center), and "M" at the Vishuddha and Ajna (throat and third-eye centers).

3. Chant the three sounds of *Om* in succession at least three times or continue chanting for as long as you like. Notice the energetic quality or qualities of the mantra as you're chanting.

4. Resting in silence with eyes closed, allow yourself to hear the inner *Om* within yourself. Give yourself at least five minutes to sit in silence, using ujjayi breath to enhance the resonance of the inner *Om*.

As you sit in meditative silence, you might begin to formulate your own description or definition of *Om* that's true for you. See if your experience and thus your definition changes over time with practice.

I see and I am released.
I am opening to wonder and expansion.
I delight in Love
and the joy of revelation.
Savoring an inner sweetness that
is "Mmm-mmm good,"
I feel connection and I understand.

Chapter 10

Practicing Perfection

Right View is not an ideology, a system, or even a
path. It is the insight we have into the reality of life, a
living insight that fills us with understanding, peace,
and love.

—Thich Nhat Hanh

I was just out of high school, beginning my first year of college,
when I walked into Professor Monte Coulter's office for my
very first drum lesson in the music department of the University
of Tennessee at Chattanooga. UTC was just a thirty-minute drive
from my parents' house in Cleveland and offered me a way to get
started with my college education, even though I wouldn't be
ready to make the leap into the big leagues at UT Knoxville until
my sophomore year. It was a convenient, cautious choice for a kid
just out of high school who wasn't really sure what he wanted to
do with his life. I knew that I loved drumming and music, that I
was good at it. Beyond that, I had no idea how I might parlay that
God-given talent into a life or even a career.

Nevertheless, I walked into Monte's office that day for my
first lesson with no shortage of confidence in my own abilities.

After all, I'd been part of an award-winning music program back home at Cleveland High School. The trophies crowded the shelves of the band room at CHS, the bounty from a learning environment where musical excellence was cultivated and expected. During my four years there, we'd won a number of national competitions for both our marching band and our jazz band. So, even as a college freshman, I already had an abundance of experience with the benefits of practice, discipline, and one-pointed focus on an ideal.

Monte and I greeted each other and he welcomed me to my first year at college. Then, before we even played a single note of music, he asked me the question that would launch my college music career. "Do you believe the saying 'Practice makes perfect'?" As someone who'd been pushed and prodded by music teachers to practice, practice, practice from the time I was eight years old, I didn't hesitate to answer, "Absolutely."

But Monte smiled and shook his head. "No, it isn't true," he said firmly. "Do you know why?" I had nothing. He looked me squarely in the eyes and said, "Because only *perfect* practice makes perfect."

I felt a little electric thrill hearing these words, sensing that he was about to usher me into a whole new and powerful approach to playing music. I had the distinct feeling that I was about to move up from the minors to the major leagues as a musician. He continued, "Think about it. Practice is just repetition, right? Over time, that repetition forms a very specific kind of physical memory in the body, like a muscle memory. Through repetition, our hands memorize the precise pattern of movement required to play a certain rhythm. Through repetition, our vocal cords memorize the exact sequence of notes required to sing a certain melody. In this way, the rhythms and melodies of music become completely ingrained in us; they become automatic and we no longer even have to consciously think about how to bring them forth. The way we've played them over and over again in our practice has been literally programmed into our body and mind.

"This is a very good thing because, as you know, when you're in the middle of a performance and the music calls for a ten-stroke roll on the snare drum, it's got to be automatic; it's got to be second nature to you. If you had to consciously think about each of those ten strokes, or where exactly to position your hands on the drum to get the right sound, or whether to start with your left hand or your right—all the little microdetails that go into that ten-stroke roll—the music would have long since passed you by and you'd be getting the evil eye from the conductor because you just missed your snare drum solo."

I smiled. This was all familiar territory for me but I sensed that Monte was about to arrive at the big insight, whatever it was that could make practice "perfect." "Now," he went on, "even though practice is an efficient and effective way to learn music, it has one very significant pitfall. Do you know what it is?"

I shook my head. "No, I really don't."

Monte handed me a pair of drumsticks. "Here, play some ten-stroke rolls for me."

On a Roll

I took the sticks in my hands and began to play the familiar pattern of one of the basic rudiments that every young drummer has to know: Right-Right-Left-Left, Right-Right-Left-Left, Right Left. The sharp sound of the snare drum echoed off the acoustic tiles of his studio and Monte watched my every move with focused attention. Thirty seconds into my little drumming demonstration, Monte held up one hand. "Okay, freeze! Keep your hands exactly where they are." My hands hovered motionless just a few inches above the white surface of the drum. "Now," he said, "look down at your hands. What do you see?"

I gazed down as I had a million times before in my years of playing and practicing the drums. Everything looked fine to me and I couldn't see any glaring problems with my grip or playing position. I shrugged a little. "Everything looks okay to me."

"What about your left hand?" he inquired. "Do you notice anything about the way you're holding the stick?" I glanced down for a closer inspection. "Are you holding the stick the same way in your left hand as in your right?" he asked.

Then it dawned on me that, compared to my right hand, my left-hand grip was somewhat collapsed at the wrist instead of maintaining a straight, clean line of energy down through the arm as it did on the right. "Hmm," I said, adjusting my left wrist ever so slightly to the proper position of alignment.

"That's it. Does your left wrist get sore or fatigued more quickly than your right?" he asked.

"Yeah, it does, actually."

"Well," he said, "that's why. Now, with that proper alignment," he went on, "let's hear some more ten-stroke rolls."

As I began to play, it took every ounce of will to keep that left hand in alignment. It felt strange, unnatural. But I could see that in this new position, my playing technique was exactly right. And I could hear the difference in the sound of the rolls. They were smoother, more even. It was a definite improvement and yet, it felt totally awkward. It was unsettling to have the technique that I could see and hear was obviously correct feel unnatural to me.

"Wow, this is really weird," I admitted, feeling shaken by

Monte's revelation. "I've been practicing this way and now it feels normal to be out of alignment."

"That's it," he said with a look of empathy. "You made a habit of misalignment without even noticing; you memorized imperfection."

Over the course of that first, one-hour lesson in Monte's studio, he patiently pointed out three significant "habits of imperfection" that I had developed unknowingly over the course of twelve years of practice. It was daunting to be faced with this trinity of imperfections in my playing, knowing that I'd have to unlearn habits that I'd been building for more than a decade. He may as well have said that I'd have to learn to walk all over again.

Sensing the despondency that was starting to take hold of me, Monte offered a helping hand. "Listen, you've got a lot of talent. These little adjustments will seem uncomfortable at first, but once you've brought everything into alignment, your playing is going to open up in ways you can't even imagine. You'll be able to play faster, smoother, and more evenly with far less effort." I nodded appreciatively, feeling a wave of optimism sweep over me.

He concluded the lesson with these words of encouragement: "From now on, when you practice, stay curious. Don't take anything for granted. Look and see and feel for yourself. Be fully aware, fully attentive, and notice everything that's happening in your body. Bring all of your energy into whatever it is that you're practicing. This way, you're not just logging hours in the practice room and, more importantly, you're not building bad habits that will cause you trouble in your playing down the road.

"You've played for long enough to know the perfect way to hold your sticks, the perfect position of your hands, wrists, and arms so that you're working *with* the laws of physics instead of against them and you're playing in the most graceful, powerful way possible. You know the perfect way to play a ten-stroke roll or any other rhythm you happen to come across. Now, to the best of your abilities, bring that perfection into everything you do on the drums. If you do this, you're practicing perfection. This way, perfection becomes your habit."

Monte wrapped up his inspiring talk with one final pearl of wisdom. "And above all, have fun with it. Enjoy the journey and be easy on yourself. When you notice that you haven't been paying full attention for a few minutes and you've allowed an old habit to creep back into your playing, just smile. Smile because you *noticed* it. Smile because you didn't let that opportunity to grow as a player pass you by. Smile because that's how you become a great musician."

That day, I left the first music lesson of my college career humbled and a little shaken. Even so, I knew there was no going back. A light switch had been turned on in my mind and now I could see a whole new dimension to this thing I'd been doing for the majority of my life. It hit home for me that day that in order for me to fully blossom as a player and as an artist, my practice had to be about quality rather than merely about quantity. I had to dedicate my attention to *how* I was practicing rather than just how much.

As I applied these new insights to my drumming practice over the weeks and months that followed, an overarching realization crystallized for me. As I began to bring more and more awareness to my practice—whether I was preparing a specific piece for performance in a concert, refining my basic drum rudiments, or working on a lesson that Monte had given me—something very profound shifted for me. The conceptual border that had existed in my mind between rehearsal and performance, between practice and music itself, started to dissolve. There was no longer this separate thing called "practice" that was somehow different from and a preparation for the real thing called "music." There was just music, even when I was practicing.

Words can't really describe how powerfully this shift transformed and enlivened my playing. My practice gradually became more and more infused with the joy, energy, and grace of a live performance. Any musician or performer knows the quality of energy that a live performance brings, the palpable electricity of a crowd engaged with rapt attention to the beauty and fullness of the moment. As I practiced, I really had the sense that the world was listening with me, that the music flowing from my hands was being shared with hundreds or thousands of eager and appreciative listeners who were enjoying this music every bit as much as I was. If you had come across me practicing in those days, you would have just seen a solitary college freshman banging away on a drum set in a drab little practice room in the music department. For me, though, the hours that I spent there behind those drums were a gateway into the Universe, into a profound connection with life and community through music.

That drum lesson with Monte all those years ago was an initiation of sorts into a powerful way of practicing music. More than that, it was really an initiation into a way of life. In the years since then, I hear echoes of Monte's teaching in the spiritual wisdom of Buddhism and Tantra.

Whether we're musicians or not, we can apply these same teachings to great effect in our meditation, chanting, and spiritual practice. One of my favorite gems of wisdom for empowering our spiritual practice is the first step of the Buddha's Eightfold Path: Right View.

The practice of mindfulness, or any other approach to meditation, only becomes an effective instrument of liberation to the extent that it is founded upon and guided by Right View.

—BHIKKHU NANAMOLI AND BHIKKHU BODHI

Samma Ditthi: Right View

After his enlightenment under the Bodhi tree, the Buddha was moved to share a method of spiritual awakening that all beings could benefit from. This method of spiritual insight handed down by the Buddha is known as the Noble Eightfold Path, symbolized by a wheel with eight spokes. This is the wheel of *dharma* (universal truth), the primary symbol of Buddhism.

The very first spoke of that wheel of dharma is *samma ditthi*, or Right View. Although the word *samma* is translated here as "right," this is not at all meant to convey anything puritanical or judgmental. There's no "Thou shalt" or "Thou shalt not" implied in Right View. If we look into the deeper meaning of this word from the ancient Pali language, we see that *samma* actually is more related to the idea of wisdom and is defined variously as "complete," "thorough," or "skillful." In addition, the Sanskrit word *samyanc*, which is sometimes used in place of *samma* to describe Right View, is defined as "same," "identical," or "united."

With these insights into the deeper meaning of this foundational teaching of the Buddha, we can see that Right View is a profound call to an embodied, lived, and felt experience in the midst of our practice—experiencing ourselves as completely united with the spiritual energies we're meditating on or chanting to.

Putting Right View Into Practice

For me, the beauty of Right View as it applies to chanting is that it calls us to enliven our practice in a very particular and powerful way; it calls us to "practice perfection." When we embrace the wisdom of Right View, we aspire to infuse every moment of our chanting practice with awareness, with heart, and, most importantly, with the felt energetic quality of whatever mantra we happen to be chanting.

When we're chanting a Lakshmi mantra to cultivate greater abundance in our lives, for example, we can cultivate the feeling-tone of Lakshmi's overflowing abundance in our hearts, in our minds, and in our bodies. We can call forth the actual felt quality of bountiful abundance right here and now in the midst of our practice. We do this by allowing ourselves to inhabit the experience that our prayers for abundance have already been answered.

As we chant those sacred sounds, which in and of themselves contain the energy of abundance, we become united with that energy, we become thoroughly steeped in the felt experience of abundance throughout our entire being. We do this through contemplation, inquiring of ourselves: What does it feel like to experience effortless abundance in our lives right now? What would that look like in our lives? How would our lives be different? How would that change the way we engage with our family, friends, community, and world? In this way, our mantra practice truly comes alive within our hearts, minds, and bodies.

Feeling the Bhav

There's a beautiful Sanskrit word that conveys this quality of practice, this state of being. *Bhava* is translated literally as "becoming," "status of being," or "state of existence." When we cultivate the feeling-tone of Lakshmi's abundance, of Shiva's wisdom, or of Saraswati's creative flow we are literally embodying those Divine archetypal energies within our own beings, we are *being* Lakshmi, Shiva, or Saraswati—we are "feeling the bhav." In this way, we are allowing the rich fullness of our mantra practice to blossom forth within us; we are steeping ourselves in the energetic qualities of our highest ideals and intentions. We are practicing perfection.

Ganesh Mantra Meditation: Clearing Obstacles with Our Inner Elephant

As an opportunity for us to experience this embodied quality of practicing perfection for ourselves, let's apply these insights to a simple but powerful mantra practice. Find a quiet place where you won't be interrupted for the next several minutes. We'll be singing along with the audio link, which you can choose to listen to through either headphones or speakers.

For this practice, we'll be chanting a mantra of Ganesh, the elephant-headed Deity who represents the clearing away of any obstacles or impediments that stand in the way of our personal or spiritual fulfillment. Before beginning this mantra meditation experience, you'll want to have chosen a particular obstacle or challenge in your life that you'd like to dedicate this practice to clearing or healing.

The mantra we'll be chanting is *Om Gam Ganapatayai Namah.* For this particular practice, we'll be singing in the powerful six-breaths-per-minute style that we read about and experienced together in the 5-Minute *Om* practice in Part One of the book. When chanting in this style, we'll take one breath between each repetition of the mantra.

You may want to warm up before the practice by either going through the "Three Priorities" vocal checklist, doing a few rounds of the Breathing Through the Universe practice, or by simply taking a few long, deep inhalations and exhalations to fill your body with breath and energy. When you're ready to begin the practice, play the audio link below and we'll get started.

Ganapati Meditation: GirishMusic.com/BookAudio

1. As you begin to chant *Om Gam Ganapatayai Namah* along with the recording, allow your voice to flow openly and freely. Sing with a full voice and sense the healing vibrations of the mantra resonating through your entire body. Notice how the sound of the mantra fills every cell of your being with its energy. Continue with this first step until you feel as though you're deeply connecting with the sound vibrations of the mantra.

2. As you continue to chant with each exhalation, with your next inhalation bring your awareness down to the sacral center at the base of the spine—known in the yogic tradition as Muladhara chakra, the abode of Ganesh. As you tune in to this primal root energy center at the base of the spine, imagine that the sound of the mantra *Om Gam Ganapatayai Namah* is emanating from here as you chant again—expanding out in all directions,

filling your entire body as well as the space around you with its healing vibrations. Then, with each new inhalation, bring your awareness again to the base of the spine, using the ujjayi breath on your inhalation to fuel the energy of your practice.

3. Continue this cycle of expanding out with the sound of the mantra, then inhaling and returning again to the root center. As you do this, sense that your energy body is growing and expanding, becoming as wide and powerful as an elephant. Stay with this part of the practice for at least the next two or three minutes until you have a palpable sense of this powerful energetic expansion within yourself.

4. Now, in this newly expanded state, allow yourself to gently bring to mind an image of the obstacle or challenge that you chose to work with in this practice. While continuing to chant and to steep in the expanded and healing energies of the practice, allow the image of the obstacle to arise in your mind almost like a photograph—keeping the experience of the mantra in the foreground of your awareness and the image of the obstacle more in the background.

5. As you continue to chant, imagine that you are directing the healing vibrations and energies of the mantra toward the image of the obstacle in your mind. You might imagine this healing energy as light pouring into the image or simply sense that the vibrations of the mantra are infusing the image as you chant. In any way that feels real for you, sense that the healing energy of *Om Gam Ganapatayai Namah* is streaming directly into the image of the obstacle—infusing and filling it—until

it gradually begins to fade from view bit by bit. Stay with this part of the practice until you have completely dissolved the image of the obstacle in your mind's eye.

6. For the final part of the practice, allow yourself to imagine and experience what your life is like now that this obstacle has been dissolved. As you continue to chant the mantra, imagine as vividly as possible what it feels like to have this obstacle cleared from your life. What's different now? What are you doing now that you couldn't do before? How does it feel? Allow yourself to steep in the feelings of this new manifestation, making it as real as you possibly can. Breathe it into yourself.

7. When you're ready for your meditation practice to come to a close, you might choose to place both hands on your heart, knowing that the healing energies you've cultivated will continue to resonate within you. As you go about your day, you can take a moment to silently repeat the mantra *Om Gam Ganapatayai Namah* to yourself, affirming the intentions of your practice anytime you choose.

Chapter 11

Finding Time to Practice

When is the best time to practice? Now.
Where is the best place to practice? Here.

It's easy sometimes to feel like there just isn't time for mantra practice, like we couldn't possibly squeeze one more thing into our already overstuffed schedules. What's more, it may be tempting to think of mantra practice as some kind of esoteric, exclusive thing that's a bit out of reach for us folks living far from the rarefied air of the Himalayan mountains from where these practices emerged. And while it's probably true that the outer circumstances of our lives look almost nothing like those of the yogis of old, the inner process—the inner journey—is exactly the same: human beings seeking the peace of the Unchanging in the midst of the changing world. It was this seeking that led ancient yogis to meditate and chant *Om* in their mountain caves, to explore and develop the very practices that we're discovering in this book. There are new singers, but the song remains the same.

Leveraging the Moment

Take a moment and do a quick mental survey of your typical day. As you're scrolling through the many activities in your little life review, take special note of the repetitive stuff that happens with minimal effort or thought on your part, as if you're moving on autopilot: filling a glass with water, brushing your teeth, making your bed, peeing, walking, driving, and on and on. Notice that there's actually a great many things we do every single day that can happen without our full, conscious participation. Our bodies assume certain positions to accomplish the task at hand, but our minds can easily be a thousand miles away.

This little insight can actually have huge implications because it shows us that, despite what we may have thought, we actually have lots of time available to us for mantra practice. We simply have to awaken to the possibility that our practice is not at all confined to any certain place or time, in the same way that our yoga asana practice doesn't end when we step off our yoga mat. In many ways, actually, it's our life off of the mat or away from the peaceful space of our home meditation room where the true practice of yoga unfolds. If we begin to leverage these countless daily moments when we might otherwise be on autopilot—transforming them into conscious opportunities for practice—we've just exponentially expanded the potential time we can invest in the yoga of chanting and, what's more, we've also infused our day-to-day existence with the inspiring, uplifting qualities of our practice.

Prayer of the Heart

When I arrived as a full-time resident at the ashram in Tennessee, it was autumn in the Smoky Mountains. In those first weeks there, I remember noticing just how fresh and crisp the mountain air felt in my lungs and how serenely quiet and peaceful it was on my nighttime walk back to my room after the evening program. In the months leading up to my first Christmas at the ashram, my teacher Shankaracharya spent many of those evening programs talking about the esoteric teachings of Christianity. He expounded on the writings of the early Christian desert fathers, the teachings of Christian mystics like Saint John of the Cross, and the Gnostic Gospels.

Having come to the ashram to immerse myself in the practices of yoga and mantra, I was definitely not expecting to spend my first few months there diving into the deeper aspects of Christianity. However, Shankaracharya clearly intended to make it his first mission with me and the other young new arrivals to reveal the threads of unity that existed between the spiritual tradition we'd come from and the one we were discovering now. I was grateful to feel that I could open to a new level of appreciation for Christianity and to discover that this yogic path I was setting out on was one of unity and oneness rather than separation or rejection.

Growing up in the church as I did, the Christian faith was familiar ground for me, but I'd certainly never encountered this decidedly different, rather yogic variety before. In the *Philokalia* (from the Greek, "Love of the Beautiful") we were introduced to the writings of the desert fathers, early Christians from between the fourth and sixth centuries who lived a monastic life in the deserts of Egypt, Palestine, and Arabia. Immersing themselves completely in a life of spiritual practice and contemplation, they sought a direct, personal experience of Spirit within their own heart, mind, and body. The details of the contemplative life these monastic Christians were living sounded quite a lot like life at the ashram, really, right down to their great affinity for a certain kind of mantra practice.

Inspired by the words of the apostle Paul in 1 Thessalonians 5:17—"Rejoice evermore" and to "pray without ceasing"—the desert fathers aspired to a form of continual spiritual practice and communion with the Divine by the constant repetition of "the Prayer of the Heart." Sometimes referred to as "the Jesus prayer" or just "the Wish," this practice of ceaseless prayer was described by the great religious scholar Huston Smith as "a Christian mantra."

Bis orat qui cantat.
(He who chants prays twice.)
—ANCIENT PROVERB

As we delved further into the details of this very yogic-sounding practice, Shankaracharya read to us from a book called *The Way of a Pilgrim*, which recounts the experiences of a nineteenth-century Russian Christian pilgrim who set out to learn how to do this Prayer of the Heart in the way of the desert fathers. In the book, the pilgrim asks for guidance from the *starets*, his spiritual teacher, who explains the practice to him this way: "The continuous interior prayer of Jesus is a constant uninter-rupted calling upon the divine name of Jesus with the lips, in the spirit, in the heart, while forming a mental picture of His constant presence, and imploring His grace, during every occupation, at all times, in all places, even during sleep."

Inspired by his teacher's words, the pilgrim sets out on his practice of the prayer, first managing to do six thousand repetitions a day and then, a few weeks later with this teacher's encouragement, twelve thousand times a day. Soon, the pilgrim finds that the joy of the prayer arises spontaneously, filling his every waking hour as effortlessly as breathing. This Prayer of the Heart is not merely an exercise in repetition, though, and the pilgrim describes how the practice revealed "the inner secret of the heart," "the knowledge of the speech of all creatures," and the direct experience of Jesus's teaching that "the kingdom of God is within you."

The ideal of returning again and again to the Prayer of the Heart was perfectly aligned with Shankaracharya's teaching that we should remember our mantra with every breath—the ajapa practice we learned about in Chapter 8, in which the mantra is repeated silently in the heart with each inhale and exhale. Even though, as dedicated yogis, we were already diving deep into mantra and meditation practice in the morning and evening programs as well as in the personal sadhana we each did on our own as part of the daily ashram routine, Shankaracharya made it clear that in many ways this ajapa mantra practice was equally if not more powerful and important than our sitting, formal practices. Engaging in this mode of moment-to-moment practice meant that our minds and hearts were steeped in the healing energy of mantra and chanting all the time, not just during those two or three hours a day of formal practice.

Shankaracharya was so keen on helping us to keep this ajapa breathing mantra practice going, he had it down to a nonverbal gesture he could employ throughout the day to remind us. He seemed to have psychic radar for when our minds had wandered off from the mantra, and he would catch our eyes and smile while silently pointing toward his heart, breathing in and out dramatically with a blissful expression on his face. Inspired by our watchful and loving teacher, we'd return once again to the sweet sound of the mantra reverberating in our hearts.

Although the original Christian practice of the Prayer of the Heart emerged from a monastic tradition, this form of moment-to-moment prayerful practice also became popular in the Eastern Orthodox Church, even among nonmonastic laypeople. In fact, even Pope John Paul II praised the advice of the desert fathers for everyone to practice the Prayer of the Heart, saying that it offered "the concrete possibility that man is given to unite himself with . . . God in the intimacy of his heart." Whether we're using a Christian prayer or a Sanskrit mantra, this unique mode of intentionally infusing every breath with sacred sound and awareness is a practice that each and every one of us can choose to benefit from.

> To live a spiritual life we must first find the courage to enter into the desert of our loneliness and to change it by gentle and persistent efforts into a garden of solitude.
> —HENRI NOUWEN

Mantra On the Go

As you begin to explore this mode of mantra on the go, try using the same mantra for both your seated, formal practice and your ajapa breath practice, particularly as you're just getting familiar with it. This sets up a powerful resonance between the deep, focused energy of your sitting practice with the more fluid, spontaneous expression of ajapa as you're moving through your day. In my experience with ajapa, I've found that the vitality and ease of the breath mantra practice is rooted in the depth of the grounded, foundational seated practice. Cultivating deep, rich experiences in the stillness of your seated mantra practice is like fertilizing the soil, allowing the dynamic flower of the breath mantra practice to blossom.

Diving deep in our seated practice also allows the particular mantra we're working with to infuse its healing vibrations more and more into our hearts and minds. Over the days and weeks, the mantra descends progressively deeper into our consciousness. This gradual encoding of the mantra's energies into our body, mind, and spirit is a process that's often described by the yogis but finds parallels in the writings of Christian mystics as well. One nineteenth-century Russian spiritual writer described the gradual unfolding of the Prayer of the Heart in three steps, which might be helpful to keep in mind in your own mantra practice:

1. **The prayer of the lips,** which is simply recitation.
2. **The focused prayer,** when the mind becomes one-pointed on the sounds of the prayer, "speaking them as if they were our own."
3. **The prayer of the heart,** "when the prayer is no longer something we do but who we are."[28]

Shankaracharya often described the same process by saying that the mantra begins at the tip of the tongue, moves to the back of the tongue, to the throat, down to the heart, and then finally the navel. Upon reaching the navel, he would say, you are no longer doing the mantra; the mantra is doing you. At that point, the energies of the mantra have become fully embodied in us.

Be mindful of this process of gradual deepening through which a mantra truly becomes integrated into our practice and our lives. Be patient with yourself, especially in the first days of working with a new mantra, trusting that, in time, it will naturally become more and more familiar and resonant for you. If you allow yourself even ten or fifteen minutes a day in the one-pointed focus of a sitting practice in front of your home altar or in your yoga room, you'll find that your mobile breath mantra practice will naturally take on a life of its own, infusing your day with the uplifting energy of your mantra.

Personally, one of my favorite mantras of all time is the *Gayatri*. I love knowing that this ancient invocation of the Light within us all has been chanted for thousands of years and that my voice joins with the voices of literally millions of others all around the world. Chanting the *Gayatri*, I feel the primal power of one of the world's great mantras and, at the same time, I feel the living connection with a global community of the heart. I've practiced the mantra formally for long periods of time, sitting in front of my altar with japa mala beads in hand, repeating those ancient syllables 108 times while meditating on the Light within me. But, I've made the *Gayatri* my mantra of choice for the ajapa breath practice as well.

I don't remember exactly when it happened, but at some point along the way the *Gayatri* became my go-to mantra for this moment-to-moment practice we've been talking about here. I go to fill a glass of water: *Om Bhur Bhuvah Svaha* ... Walking to the store: *Tat Savitur Varenyam* ... Time to pee: *Bhargo Devasya Dhimahi* ... Lying in bed as I drift off to sleep: *Dhiyo Yo Nah Pracho-*

dayaat. In this way, there are little glimpses of Light all through the day, not just when I'm sitting formally in front of the altar.

As you begin to mine your daily life for little gems of practice opportunity, the very best mantra for you to use is the one that speaks to you, the one that resonates with you, the one you feel a heart connection with. It often happens that the mantra we're practicing in formal Sadhana naturally bubbles up throughout the day of its own accord. As I mentioned earlier, this is a beautiful way to continue deepening your connection with the mantra and to bask in the energy even as you go about your life.

But there are really no rules, especially once you've been working with the breath practice for a while. If another mantra comes to mind and it feels right, just go with it. As you learn more about the beautiful and diverse world of mantra energies, you may find that a certain mantra arises that is perfectly suited to support you in whatever is happening in your life right now. Remember, all the Deities are simply expressions of Divine qualities already within you. Trust the innate knowing within you to guide you on your journey.

As you embark on this journey of mantrafying your breath throughout the day, will you find your entire being suddenly bathed in white light while standing in line at the supermarket? Possibly. Will radiant streams of cosmic insight pour into your mind as you fill a glass with water? It could happen. But, with or without these cosmic fireworks, there is one certainty about leveraging the moment in this way: when we choose the alternative of engaging consciously in our mantra practice rather than returning unconsciously to habitual mental chatter, we are, without a doubt, giving ourselves the very real gift of a more uplifting, more expansive, more peaceful, and more loving experience in that very moment.

Whichever mantra comes to you easily and spontaneously is the one you should do. It should give a strong feeling and be like music flowing from the heart.

—MOTHER MEERA

Bringing It All Together: Creating Your Own Daily Mantra Practice

Finding the inspiration to practice every day is the living heart of the yoga of chanting. As we've seen in this chapter, our practice need not be confined only to a cross-legged position in a certain room of our house. We can turn to our mantra again and again through the course of our entire day, taking our practice on the road, sometimes literally. In seeking to keep the fire of our mantra practice burning, it's helpful to draw from many different styles and modes of chanting. Kirtan, japa, likhita, ajapa, stotram, and chalisa: these unique and various modes of the yoga of chanting offer us a wealth of inspiration to fuel our mantra practice.

When we're ready to embrace a daily mantra practice of some kind, we'll want to begin by choosing a mantra that really resonates with us, one that we sense a special connection with. We want to feel as though we've found the perfect mantra for us right now; one that aligns with whatever intention brought us to the practice in the first place. Keep in mind that you are the only one who will know which mantra is right for you. Just listen to your heart and go with your instinct.

If you'd like a little inspiration, you could simply peruse the wide variety of mantras in the Songbook for the Soul section of the book. There, you'll find dozens of mantras along with clear explanations of the traditional uses and qualities of each. Or perhaps you'll feel a special affinity for the image or the energetic qualities of Ganesh, Lakshmi, Hanuman, Shakti, and Shiva as you're reading the inspiring stories and insights associated with these Deities. You might try gently holding the thought of your intention in mind as you look through the mantras in the Songbook, to see if something clicks. When it's right, you'll know it.

To get a feel for what a daily mantra practice might look like, I'll share a simple but powerful practice—one that combines the elements of mindful singing that we learned in Part One with the japa mantra practice we learned in Part Two. As you'll see, the beauty of this combination is in how the mindful singing opens and attunes us for an even deeper experience with the japa mantra that comes after it.

For this practice, we'll be using the mantra *Om Namah Shivaya* for both the mindful singing as well as the japa practice. Keep in mind, you can use this mindful singing/japa combination with any other mantras you might choose. Once you get the hang of it, you'll see how you can get creative with this kind of practice to fuel your daily mantra immersion.

Find a quiet place where you won't be disturbed for the next ten minutes or so. We'll be using the audio link for the first part of the practice, and you'll want to have headphones or speakers ready so you can sing along. You'll also want to have a japa mala, or rosary, for the second half of the practice.

For the first part of the practice, we'll be singing in the powerful six-breaths-per-minute style that we read about and experienced together in the 5-Minute *Om* practice in Part One of the book. When chanting in this style, we'll take one breath between each word of the *Om Namah Shivaya* mantra.

You may want to warm up before the practice by either going through the "Three Priorities" vocal checklist, doing a few rounds of the Breathing Through the Universe practice, or by simply taking a few long, deep inhalations and exhalations to fill your body with breath and energy. When you're ready to begin the practice, play the audio link below and we'll get started.

Om Namah Shivaya: GirishMusic.com/BookAudio

1. As you begin to chant *Om Namah Shivaya* along with the recording, allow your voice to flow openly and freely. Sing with a full voice and sense the healing vibrations of the mantra resonating through your entire body. Notice how the sound of the mantra fills every cell of your being with its energy. Connect with the support of your inner flowerpot (see Chapter 5) as you sing so that your voice can sustain comfortably.

2. Continue to sing the mantra along with the recording until it gradually fades after about six minutes. As the sound of the recording begins to grow quieter, allow your own voice to get softer, too, until it's almost a whisper.

3. Now, as you release the external chanting of the mantra, take your japa mala in hand and begin to recite *Om Namah Shivaya* within yourself. In this part of the practice, you can relinquish the melody of the chant, simply allowing the pure sound vibrations of *Om Namah Shivaya* to arise naturally and spontaneously within you as each mala bead passes over your fingers. Go at your own pace so that you can savor each repetition of the

mantra. Use ujjayi breath to enhance the resonance of the mantra within you.

4. Once you've reached the meru bead on your mala, you might choose to continue by reversing the mala in your hand and continuing around again in this way for as long as you like.

5. When you've reached the end of your final round of malas and you feel complete, simply return to your natural breath and allow yourself to take in the energy you've generated in your practice. Breathe this healing energy into yourself fully and take it in.

6. When you feel complete, place both hands on your heart knowing that you carry the energies of your practice with you as you carry on with your day.

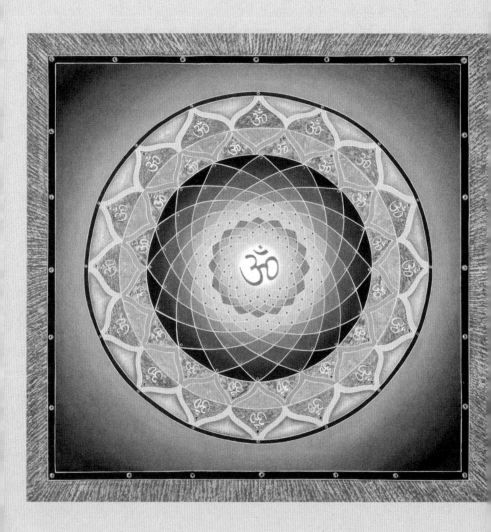

PART THREE

Songbook for the Soul

Chapter 12

Sanskrit:
Our Divine Heritage

I am convinced that everything has come down to us
from the banks of the Ganges.

—Voltaire

All the mantras in the Songbook for the Soul come to us from the ancient Sanskrit language: the "language of the Gods." First appearing in the writings of the *Vedas*, India's oldest scriptures, dating back at least three thousand years, Sanskrit is held in high regard as one of the world's great sacred languages. From the perspective of the wisdom traditions of India, Sanskrit is the original language of the perennial Hindu classics including the *Vedas, Upanishads, Bhagavad Gita, and Ramayana,* among many others. In other words, Sanskrit has massive street cred in terms of its ability to deliver the spiritual goods.

Sanskrit also has two other qualities to be mindful of as we endeavor to bravely leap into new and unknown chanting territory. The first quality is that Sanskrit is said to be an "intrinsic" language. In other words, the term for any given thing in Sanskrit is not an arbitrary symbol but, rather, contains the intrinsic nature of the thing itself. So, if we're chanting a Ganesh mantra, the sound isn't just a name for Ganesh, it *is* Ganesh himself in vibrational form—Ganesh's sound body. The mantra *is* the Deity. As my teacher Shankaracharya liked to say, "The sound and the meaning are one."

A quick story about this intrinsic quality of sound: During my second year at the ashram, a Brahmin priest from Sri Lanka named Haran Aiya came out to stay with us for a few days and to perform a beautiful activation ceremony for our *Shiva Lingam* (a symbolic representation of Lord Shiva). At one point in the festivities, Haran told us the story of his days as a boy, learning by heart the many incredibly long and complicated chants, scriptures, and invocations required for his coming life as a priest in the Divine Mother tradition. According to that tradition, a young, aspiring priest would learn the chants by listening to the elder priest, memorizing and repeating it back with utmost precision. However, Haran explained, no translations whatsoever were given for these chants—only the proper pronunciation, melody, and cadence. So, from the time he was five or six until he was twelve, he was taught in this way, immersing himself purely in the sounds of the mantras and chanting day after day.

When Haran finally turned twelve, the elder priests celebrated his coming of age with a big ceremony in which they finally revealed the meanings of all these elaborate chants that he'd been memorizing for the past several years. "But," Haran explained, "these translations were no revelation for me at all. I already knew the meanings perfectly! Why? Because the Divine Mother herself had explained every single word to me as I was chanting them."

We can experience this intrinsic quality of mantra for ourselves, in the laboratories of our own bodies. For example, Chapter 9, "The Three Sounds of Om," is an in-depth exploration of the mantra *Om* with a simple, three-step practice that will open us to an experience of this self-contained wisdom of sound.

There's a second quality we can notice about Sanskrit that can support us in feeling more comfortable and confident in our journey through the wide world of mantra. It may be surprising to discover that, whether we've ever chanted a single mantra before in our lives, if our native tongue happens to be English, Spanish, French, German, Russian, Portuguese, or any one of the nearly 450 Indo-European dialects—Sanskrit is, in fact, the likely root from which the branch of our native language has sprouted. This means that we're already using many words with Sanskrit roots every single day!

Let's do a little experiment to see how this might support us in finding our way around the Sanskrit language. Before reading the Sanskrit Root Words list on the next page, find a small blank piece of paper. Now, cover up the column of English words on the right.

Begin by reading the first Sanskrit word on the left. Read it over and sound it out to yourself a couple of times either out loud or in your head. Focus primarily on the actual sound of the word, rather than the spelling. Does it sound familiar in any way? Does it remind you of some other word? Now, uncover the corresponding English word on the right side and see how you did. Go through the entire list like this, one line at a time.

A couple of quick pronunciation tips:

    a = "u," as in *but*
    aa = "a," as in *father*
    i = "ee," as in *see*

SANSKRIT ROOT WORDS

ROOT SANSKRIT WORD	DERIVED ENGLISH WORD
Braathra	Brother
Danta	Dental
Dwar	Door
Harda	Heart
Jangala	Jungle
Loka	Locale/Location
Madhyam	Medium
Manu	Man
Matar	Mother
Naam	Name
Na	No
Navagatha	Navigation
Ritam	Rhythm
Sama	Same
Tat	That
Thri	Three

How did you do? Most people are surprised at how often their "guesses" are correct. But even if you were only able to see the correlation between these words after uncovering both sides of the list, still, what does that tell you?

While this is by no means a comprehensive list of all the words that have been derived from the Sanskrit language—not to mention the straight-out Sanskrit terms that we've adopted unchanged ("political *pundits*," "tech *gurus*," "good *karma*")—it demonstrates a powerful principle that we can return to again and again in our chanting adventures: the ancient Sanskrit dialect is in some ways already familiar to us because it's very likely that many of the words in our own language came from Sanskrit in the first place. And this is true for the majority of people around the world, because the Indo-European languages are the native tongue of some three billion people, the largest by far of any known language group.

As you travel through the wide world of Sanskrit chanting, be on the lookout for words that seem somehow familiar—you might just be getting in touch with your own inner Sanskrit scholar! If we can be mindful of both the intrinsic wisdom inherent within the sound as well as our deep linguistic connection with the Sanskrit language, then we will deepen and expand our own experience dramatically.

To help get you started on your mantra and chanting adventure, here's a list of frequently used Sanskrit words, what I call bits of mantra DNA, that can give a hint to the mantra's purpose.

Om: the sound of the experience of Oneness

Maha: great

Shakti: the Divine feminine

Para or *Param*: supreme, transcendent

Sarva or *Sarvam*: all, everything

Devi or *Deva*: feminine or masculine Divinity, respectively, literally "shining one"

Shiva: the Divine masculine, the bliss of consciousness, literally "the auspicious one"

Rupa or *Rupam*: form, appearance

Jaya or *Jay* or *Jai*: victory, may it be victorious

Shri: holy

Ananda: bliss, joy

Hare or *Hari*: the energy of God, remover of illusions

Swaha or *Svaha*: oblations, let it be so

All of the mantras and chants in the following songbook chapters have been written out in such a way that they will resemble regular English pronunciation with only a few exceptions. This style of transliteration allows us easier access to the sounds of the chants without the need for diacritical marks that might be confusing.

Here are the six pronunciation exceptions to keep an eye out for as you're going through the mantras in the Songbook for the Soul:

a = "u" as in *hut*

aa = "a" as in *father*

ai = "ai" as in *aisle*

au = "ou" as in *sound*

e = "ay" as in *hay*

i (at the end of a word) = "ee" as in *see*

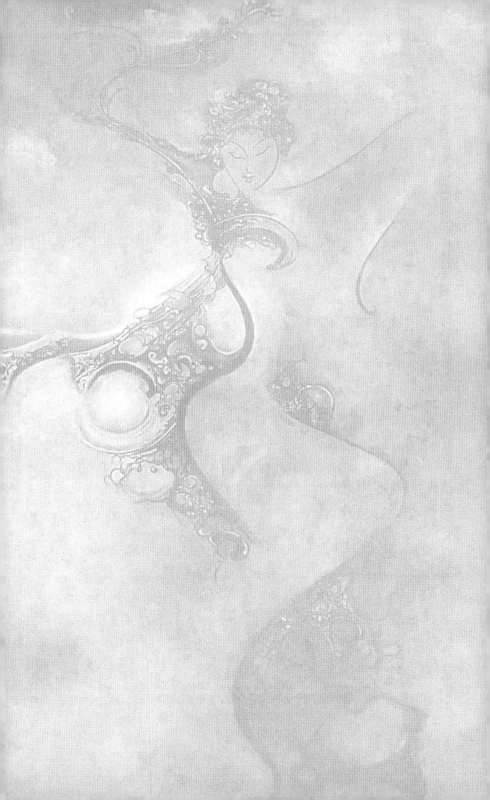

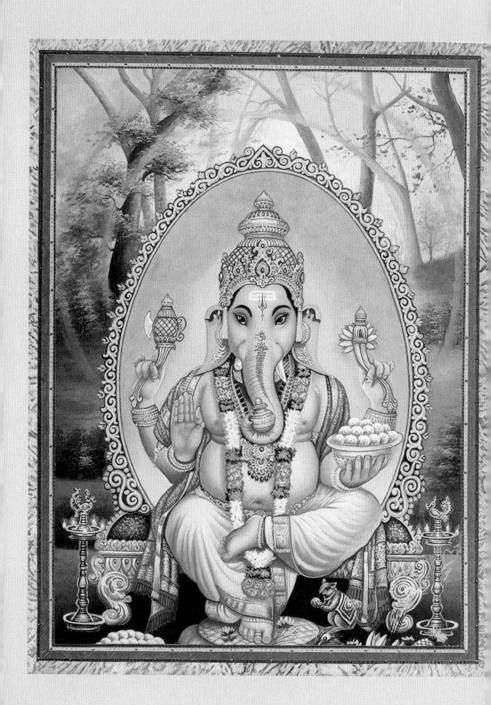

Chapter 13

Ganesh Mantras

The elephant-headed Deity named Ganesh is one of the most recognizable icons in the pantheon of Hindu Gods and Goddesses. Images and statues of him can be seen adorning the walls of Indian establishments all around the world. This is a testament to Ganesh's role as the remover of obstacles, clearing the way for success in earthly life. He is known as "the First" and the "Lord of beginnings," affirming his role as the first Divine archetype to be invoked to ensure success in all endeavors.

The name Ganesh or Ganesha comes from two Sanskrit root words: *gana*, meaning "multitude" or "category," and *isha*, meaning "Lord" or "Ruler." In one sense, he represents the unity of all life and all existence, the common thread of consciousness that connects all the vast realms of existence.

Like all the Gods and Goddesses of Hinduism, Ganesh has many names, which reveal the archetypal qualities he embodies. For instance, he's known as Vakratunda, "he who straightens out the crooked," or Buddhipriya, "he who loves wisdom." He's sometimes referred to as Anantachidrupamayam, "the infinite and consciousness personified," or Omkara, "the embodiment of *Om*."

He's also called Ekadanta, which literally means "one-tusked," re-ferring to the fact that he is always pictured with just a single tusk, signifying his embodiment of wisdom beyond duality—Oneness. The single tusk also refers to the ideal of one-pointedness and *pratyahara*, gathering up and focusing our sometimes scattered energies through the practices of yoga so that we can "go big." In this way, I sometimes think of Ganesh as a kind of magnifying glass through which the diverse rays of our own light are gathered up into a powerful, one-pointed coherence. Through Ganesh, we light the transformative fire of yoga within ourselves.

Beyond the traditional teachings about Ganesh, what does the energetic archetype embodied in his colorful form really represent for us in our mantra practice and in our lives? One clue can be found in the common notion that Ganesh's abode is said to be the Muladhara chakra—the sacral center at the base of our spine. This suggests that Ganesh can be seen as being intimately con-nected with the primal spiritual energy called *kundalini*, which the yogis tell us resides at the base of the spine. When this massively powerful and transformative energy awakens, the karmic obsta-cles in our lives are naturally burned away. In this way, Ganesh represents the calling to a life of true yoga and spiritual practice, one in which we cultivate a living experience of our Divine nature.

Putting aside mythology for a moment, when we look at Ga-nesh's image we can plainly see a human being who has somehow undergone a radical transformation. We see a rather portly-bellied person with various items in hand and . . . what's this? The head of an elephant? The famous story of how Ganesh got his elephant head honestly never resonated much for me—that is, until I learned an esoteric interpretation of the popular tale, which I'll share in a moment.

First, in the common telling of the Ganesh mythology, the Divine Mother, Parvati, wants to take a bath whilst her beloved Shiva is away. Since there is no one else there to stand guard to make sure that her bath is undisturbed, she simply takes a bit of her own skin and, breathing life into it, creates a Divine being—Ganesh—right on the spot, instructing him to forbid anyone from disturbing her watery retreat. After some time, however, Shiva returns and is none too pleased when this Ganesh fellow refuses him entrance to Parvati's presence. With continued resistance from the tenacious Ganesh, Shiva resorts to cutting off his head. Meanwhile, Parvati comes out from her bath to see what all the commotion is about. Highly annoyed that Shiva has dispatched her Divine offspring, she informs him of Ganesh's identity as her creation and insists that Shiva rectify this situation immediately. In a flash, Shiva commands his servants to go and fetch him the head of the first creature they find sleeping while facing in a northerly direction. The servants look high and low but can't find anyone sleeping in that particular direction other than . . . you guessed it, an elephant. But Shiva, being the "Great God," just worked with what he had and brought Ganesh back to life, elephant head and all. Ta-da!

Diving deep below the surface of this story to a more esoteric understanding of the Ganesh mythology, Parvati as Shakti represents the Divine energy of kundalini within us all. Her bath represents the cleansing and purifying effect of yoga and spiritual practice. In this version of the story, Ganesh first appears representing the protective shield of ego, the sense of individuality. Once the process of purification is complete, however, true wisdom arrives in the form of Lord Shiva destroying the illusion of ego and separation. With the small, individual ego dissolved in the light of wisdom, Shiva replaces it with the universal ego in the form of the big elephant head, meaning that we no longer identify only with our individual self but with the universal Self of all. In this version of the tale, Ganesh has in some ways become the picture of a Divine human, fully experiencing his or her spiritual nature.

In our journey with mantra practice, Ganesh can be seen as our home base, the energetic foundation upon which we can build by gathering up our energy and light through the practices of yoga and chanting. In particular, if we're just beginning a mantra practice for the first time, a Ganesh mantra is the best place to start. The energy of Ganesh is about clearing away obstacles and impediments in our path so that success, abundance, and spiritual growth can blossom in our lives.

Ganesh Mantras

The following mantras are best suited for japa mala practice. You can hear the pronunciation of the following mantras in the audio link below.

Ganesh Mantras 1–8: GirishMusic.com/BookAudio

1. Om Gam Ganapatayai Namah
The primary Ganesh mantra for clearing obstacles and awakening the primal root energy of consciousness. Translated as "Salutations to the remover of obstacles," the mantra contains Ganesh's seed-sound "Gam." This mantra can be used before any new endeavor or event. It also prepares us for the attainment of personal power and assists the purification of the ego. Located at the base of the spine where the Kundalini Shakti resides, Ganesh merges masculine and feminine, power and wisdom, the ongoing forces of our individual evolution.

2. Om Shri Ganeshaaya Namah

This mantra is said to enhance the power of the mind and memory. It removes obstacles—both internal and external—to success, prosperity, and knowledge.

3. Om Lambodharaaya Namah

A mantra to invoke the experience of Oneness with the Universe, bringing harmony and peace by allowing us to assimilate all experiences—both good and bad. The mantra is translated as "Salutations to the big-bellied one." Ganesh is said to hold the entire Universe in his belly, allowing us to connect to the universal energy through his mantra. This mantra is also said to give us the ability to accumulate and store vast knowledge.

4. Om Vakratundaaya Hum

A mantra for clearing negativities, both internal and external. Vakratunda refers to Ganesh's power of straightening out whatever is not in alignment. The translation of the mantra is, "Salutations to he with twisted trunk, removing negativity with the weapon mantra Hum." This mantra can be used when things are not working properly to straighten them out, individually or universally. It releases negativity in oneself or others on all levels, physical, emotional, mental, and spiritual.

5. Om Ekadantaaya Namah

A mantra to invoke a one-pointed state of mind that can achieve anything through devotion. The mantra means, "Salutations to he with one tusk," and it can assist us in choosing one aim and traveling toward it for success.

This mantra facilitates looking beyond duality and moving ahead single-mindedly in life without doubts or distractions.

6. Om Shreem Hreem Kleem Glaum Gam Ganapatayai Namah

A powerful mantra to invoke the energies of abundance into our lives by clearing away all energetic obstacles and cultivating the energy of attracting our highest good. The mantra can be translated as, "Salutations to the remover of obstacles," and it is enhanced with the seed-sounds of Lakshmi (Shreem), Mahamaya (Hreem), the principle of attraction (Kleem), as well as two seed-sounds for Ganesh, embodying the principles of will and focused power. This is a mantra to help with the removal of obstacles, to attract abundance, to clear away illusion, and bring forth the experience of our inner Divinity through the grace of Ganesh.

7. Om Ucchista Ganapatayai Namah

A mantra that is said to destroy negativities and karmic obstacles. The mantra can be translated as, "Salutations to the Dark Ganesh, destroying all evil." You can visualize Ganesh dark in color while chanting this mantra to destroy all negativities both inside and out.

8. Om Shreem Gam Ganapataye Namah

A mantra for prosperity that combines Lakshmi's energy of abundance with the obstacle-removing energy of Ganesh. The mantra can be translated as, "Salutations to Ganesh," enhanced with the added seed-sound of

Lakshmi, "Shreem." This mantra is said to remove any obstacles to the flowering of abundance.

Ganesh Gayatri Mantra

Ganesh *Gayatri* Mantra: GirishMusic.com/BookAudio

Om Ekadantaaya Vidmahe
Vakratundaaya Dheemahi
Tanno Dantih Prachodayaat

This is a powerful meditation mantra that is said to invoke an experience of unity with all of creation and to facilitate the dawning of spiritual enlightenment through the grace of Ganesh. The mantra may be translated as, "We pray to the one with the single-tusk who is omnipresent. We meditate upon and pray for greater intellect to the Lord with the curved, elephant-shaped trunk. We bow before the one with the single-tusk to illuminate our minds with wisdom."[29]

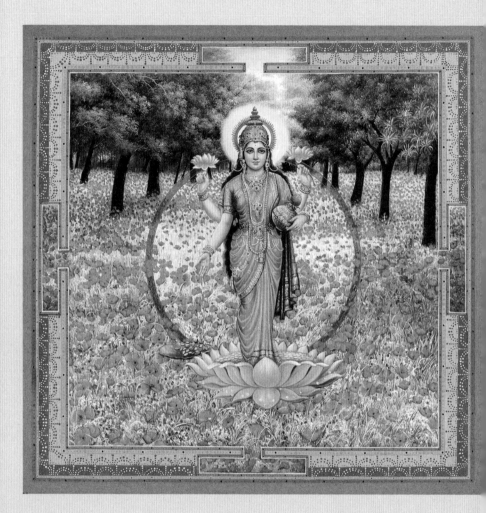

Chapter 14

Lakshmi Mantras

I f Ganesh could be said to be the sacred foundation of earth we cultivate through the practices of yoga, the goddess Lakshmi is like a radiant, beautiful flower blossoming from that sanctified ground. She is known as the Goddess of wealth, success, and fortune, but as with all the Divine archetypes, she is much more than the particular qualities she embodies. Lakshmi, like all the other Deities, is a window into the Infinite, into Oneness.

As the Shakti or energy of Vishnu, the Hindu Deity who is said to sustain and protect the Universe, Lakshmi embodies the auspicious qualities of prosperity, royal power, success, and illustriousness. She represents not only financial abundance, but an abundance of anything we value in life: love, good health, harmonious relationships, peace, and more. She is pictured as a stunningly beautiful Goddess dressed in radiant red atop a blooming pink lotus flower, surrounded by two regal elephants. Her four arms represent the attainment of the four goals of life: *dharma* (Right Living), *kama* (pleasure, fulfillment of desires), *artha* (spiritual and material wealth), and *moksha* (liberation from birth and death). Her front hands with golden coins streaming forth show her bestowing earthly riches, while her two back hands hold aloft two lotus flowers, indicating her blessings of spiritual attainment.

The image of the lotus is often associated with Lakshmi, as many of her other names reveal. She is known as Kamalasambhava, "originating from the lotus," Padmasundari, "one who is as beautiful as a lotus," Padma, "lotus-dweller," Padmapriya, "one who loves lotuses," and Padmamaladhara Devi, "one who wears a garland of lotuses," among many others.

Lakshmi's association with the image of the lotus can be seen to express two primary qualities embodied in this beloved Goddess. First, the lotus represents the abundant fertility of earthly life, flowering forth in all its creative expression. Here, we see Lakshmi's well-known attributes of overflowing success and prosperity in worldly endeavors. However, the lotus conveys a deeper, spiritual meaning as well and is seen as a symbol of exalted spiritual attainment and realization. Although rooted in the mud below, the unstained lotus blossoms beautifully above the water, conveying a transcendent spiritual state that has risen above mere material concerns. In the image of Lakshmi, we see the embodiment of both earthly and spiritual attainment.

The blossoming lotus of Lakshmi's energetic presence in our lives unfolds in the Anahata chakra, the heart center in the middle of the chest that is said to embody the union and balance of male and female energies within us. In one of the earliest known chants to Lakshmi, the ancient Vedic hymn called the *Shri Suktam*, the Goddess of abundance is said to reside in the heart:

Padme-sthitaam Padma-varnaam
*Seated in the heart center, Your grandeur resembles a
lotus in full bloom.*

Elsewhere in the hymn, she is expressed as the mother of love itself, embodied in her son Chiklita:

Aapah Srijantu Snigdhaani Chiklita Vasa Me Grihe
Ni Cha Deveem Maataram Shriyam Vaasaya Me Kule
May the waters of love pour forth resplendently. O God
of Love, may your presence reveal your brilliant mother,
Lakshmi, within my heart.

These and many other verses in various chants convey the insight that Lakshmi represents the awakened, loving energy of our own heart. Once we've risen above the self-centered desires of our lower nature, our life-energy is free to blossom from our hearts in the form of love, compassion, and healing; we are free to follow our true heart's calling.

As you chant these sacred sounds and mantras of Lakshmi, allow your awareness to dwell in the Anahata chakra, where we can experience our connection with our higher nature as love itself. Place your left hand over the center of your chest and feel the vibrations of the mantra within yourself. Allow the lotus of your heart to blossom with every breath.

Lakshmi Mantras

The following mantras are best suited for japa mala practice. You can hear the pronunciation of the following mantras in the audio link below.

Lakshmi Mantras 1–4: GirishMusic.com/BookAudio

1. Om Shreem Shreeyai Namah

A mantra invoking Lakshmi's creative abundance in all its forms. It can be translated as, "Salutations to the primal all-pervading energy." This mantra may be chanted to bring abundance and attune with the primordial feminine energy.

2. Om Shreem Shreem Shreem Mahaa Lakshmyai Namah

This variation of the MahaLakshmi *mantra amps up the energy of the seed-sound "Shreem," and increases the energy of creative abundance within us. It can be translated as, "Salutations to that heart-centered and great Lakshmi," enhanced with the added power of Lakshmi's seed-sound "Shreem." This mantra may be used to attune to the Goddess Lakshmi's energy for abundance—both spiritual and material—health, and prosperity in all forms.*

3. Om Hreem Shreem Lakshmibhyo Namah

A mantra for attaining wealth and prosperity, adding the seed-sound "Hreem," which adds the energy of Divine attraction. Said to open the heart, this mantra is chanted to bestow blessings of abundance in all aspects of one's life through the grace of Lakshmi. It is particularly good for calling in abundance that is in line with our soul's purpose or true calling.

4. Om Lakshmi Ganapatayai Namah

A mantra for prosperity that combines Lakshmi's energy of abundance with the obstacle-removing energy of

Ganesh. This mantra is said to remove any obstacles to the flowering of abundance.[30]

Mahaalakshmyashtakam Hymn

The *Mahaalakshmyashtakam* is a beautiful hymn to Lakshmi that emphasizes her deeper meaning as the embodiment of the primal, all-pervading creative energy, which manifests as overflowing abundance—both material and spiritual. You'll find the recorded version of this text chant in the audio link.

Mahaalakshmyashtakam: **GirishMusic.com/BookAudio**

1. **Namaste'stu Mahaamaaye Shreepeethe Surapoojite Shankha chakra gadaa haste Mahaalakshmi Namo'stu Te**

    Salutations to Thee, great Enchantress. You are the source of good fortune, worshipped by the gods. You bear the conch of creative vibration, the discus of revolving time and the mace which subdues negativities. O Mahaalakshmi, we salute Thee.

2. **Namaste Garudaaroodhe Kolaasura bhayankari Sarva paapa hare Devi Mahaalakshmi Namo'stu Te**

    Salutations to Thee, rider of the wings of speech, terrorizer of egoism and conqueror of imperfection. O beloved Mahaalakshmi, we salute Thee.

3. **Sarvajne Sarvavarade Sarva dushta bhayankari**
   Sarva duhkha hare Devi Mahaalakshmi Namo'stu Te
   You are the knower of everything, bestower of boons,
   vanquisher of corruption and remover of all misery. O
   beloved Mahaalakshmi, we salute Thee.

4. **Siddhi buddhi prade Devi Bhukti mukti pradaayini**
   Mantra moorte Sadaa Devi Mahaalakshmi Namo'stu Te
   O Goddess, ever manifesting as the mantra, You bestow
   discrimination, good fortune, worldly pleasure and
   enlightenment. O beloved Mahaalakshmi, we salute
   Thee.

5. **Aadyanta rahite Devi Aadyashakti Maheshvari**
   Yogaje Yogasambhoote Mahaalakshmi Namo'stu Te
   O Goddess, You are beyond time, primordial and
   begotten of yoga. O great mistress Mahaalakshmi, we
   salute Thee.

6. **Sthoola sookshma mahaaraudre Mahaashakti Mahodare**
   Mahaa paapa hare Devi Mahaalakshmi Namo'stu Te
   Taking form in gross and subtle bodies, You are the
   Shakti of Rudra, the origin of everything and the
   expeller of sins. O beloved Mahaalakshmi, we salute
   Thee.

7. **Padmaasana sthite Devi Parabrahma svaroopini**
   Parameshi Jagan maatar Mahaalakshmi Namo'stu Te
   O Goddess, reposed upon a lotus, You are the
   embodiment of Brahman, the supreme mistress. O
   Mahaalakshmi, Mother of the worlds, we salute Thee.

8. **Shvetaambaradhare Devi Naanaalankara bhooshite**
Jagat sthite Jagan maatar Mahaalakshmi Namo'stu Te

> *O Goddess, dressed in white and ornamented with the*
> *finest jewels, You are the sustainer of the cosmos and the*
> *Mother of all the worlds. O beloved Mahaalakshmi, we*
> *salute Thee.*[31]

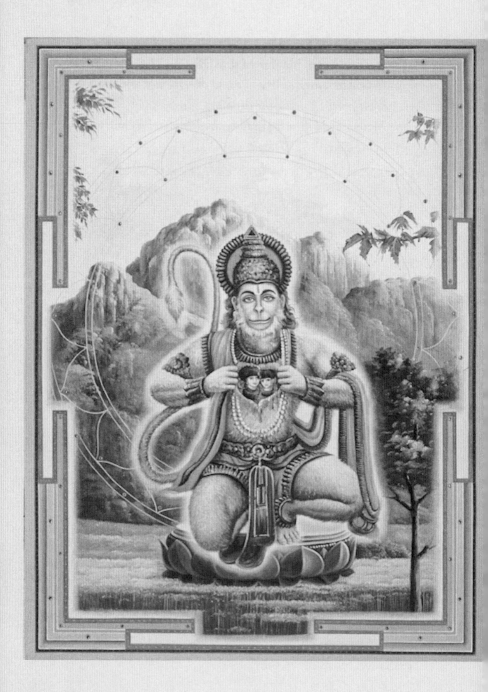

Chapter 15

Hanuman Mantras

Hanuman is the embodiment of supreme selfless devotion, strength, courage, humility, and the powerful spiritual vitality that arises from a life lived in service to a higher ideal. In the context of yoga and the spiritual path, he represents the ideal of leading with the Heart. The Divine archetype of Hanuman inspires us to put Love first, living from the Heart rather than the head.

In his mythological incarnation in the great spiritual epic the *Ramayana*, Hanuman appears as a leader of the Vanaras, a race of beings who were half man, half monkey. However, Hanuman is no mere primate. Through a boon bestowed to his parents by Brahma and the other gods, Hanuman is endowed with all the yogic powers, or *siddhis*. His name is said to derive from the well-known story of his childhood when he leapt up to the sun, thinking it was an orange he could gobble up, incurring a blow from Indra's thunderbolt that broke his jaw. Thus, his name comes from the Sanskrit roots *hanu*, which means "jaw," and *mant*, which means "broken" or "disfigured." His namesake and the story of this early, formative experience reveals one of his most essential characteristics: humility and the absence of ego.

This rare combination of Divine power and humility inspired Rama, an incarnation of Vishnu, to enlist Hanuman as his messenger. It's in this role of Rama's emissary that Hanuman achieves his heroic status, reuniting the Divine King, Rama, with his beloved consort, Sita, who has been kidnapped by the evil Ravana. Of course, behind the colorful mythology we find a deeper meaning, one that speaks to our own spiritual journey.

Our first clue to this inner meaning of the famous story can be found in one of Hanuman's other names, Maruti, which means "born of the wind." Hanuman's father, in fact, is Vayu, the "breath of Life" and the embodiment of prana. This identification of Hanuman with prana reveals that his one-pointed devotion to Lord Rama can be seen as symbolizing the path of controlling and cultivating our own pranic energies through yogic practices such as mantra, chanting, pranayama, and meditation.

In the same way, the reuniting of Rama and Sita—the crowning moment of Hanuman's story as told in the *Ramayana*—can be seen as symbolic of the culmination of our own spiritual journey. In this deeper vision of the tale, Rama represents our Higher Self, while Sita represents the intuitive wisdom or *buddhi*, the higher faculty of the mind that allows us to perceive our spiritual nature. Ravana can be seen as representing the ego, obscuring our perception of our Higher Self. Hanuman, as the embodiment of life-energy cultivated through the practice of yoga, is the bridge that reunites the Divine couple.

As you chant these sacred sounds and mantras of Hanuman, allow your breath to enhance the experience of vital, pranic energy flowing into your body, filling you with love, strength, courage, fearlessness, and confidence rooted in your connection with your Higher Self.

Hanuman Mantras

The following mantras are best suited for japa mala practice. You can hear the pronunciation of the following mantras in the audio link below.

Hanuman Mantras 1–3: GirishMusic.com/BookAudio

1. **Om Shree Hanumaate Namah**

   A Hanuman mantra invoking strength, stamina, and power. The mantra can be translated as, "Salutations to Hanuman, the embodiment of awakened pranic energy."

2. **Om Ham Hanumaate Namah**

   This mantra adds the power of Hanuman's seed-sound "Ham" which conveys protection, removal of negativities, strength, and wisdom.

3. **Om Ham Hanumaate Rudraatmakaaya Hum Phat Svaahaa**

   A powerful Hanuman mantra that adds the illusion-dissolving wisdom energy of Shiva and the seed-sounds "Hum" (invoking the inner fire to burn away negativities) and "Phat" (an emphatic, explosive cutting away of negativities). Swami Satyananda Saraswati translates this mantra as, "Om. We bow to the Highest Principle, to Hanumaan, the manifestation of the Reliever of Sufferings (Shiva). Cut the Ego! Purify! I am one with God!"[32]

Hanuman Chalisa

The *Hanuman Chalisa*, with over forty stanzas, is undoubtedly the most well-known chant to Hanuman. It was composed by the fifteenth-century poet-saint Tulsidas, who was considered to be one of the greatest Indian literary figures. Tulsidas also wrote the famous poetic retelling of the *Ramayana* called the *Ramcharitmanas*. You'll find the recorded version of this text chant in the audio link.

Hanuman Chalisa: GirishMusic.com/BookAudio

1. **Bhajelo Ji Hanumaan! Bhajelo Ji Hanumaan!**
   O Friend! Sing the praises of Hanuman!

2. **Shree Guru charana saroja raja,**
   Nija manu mukuru sudhaari
   Having polished the mirror of my heart with the dust on my Guru's lotus feet.

3. **Baranaun Raghubara bimala jasu,**
   Jo daayaku phala chaari
   I sing the pure fame of the best of the Raghus, which bestows the Four Fruits of Life.

4. **Bhudhi heena tanu jaanike,**
   Sumiraun pavana kumaara
   Knowing this body to be devoid of intelligence, I recall the Son of the Wind.

5. **Bala budhi vidya dehu mohin,**
   Harahu kalesa bikaara

   Grant me strength, wit and wisdom, and remove my
   sorrows and shortcomings.

6. **Seeyaavara Raamachandra pada Jai Sharanam**

   Hail the refuge of the feet of Sita's bridegroom,
   Ramachandra.

7. **Jaya Hanumaana gyaana guna saagara,**
   Jaya Kapeesha tihun loka ujaagara

   Victory to Hanuman, ocean of wisdom and virtue.
   Hail Monkey Lord, illuminator of the three
   worlds.

8. **Raama doota atulita bala dhaamaa,**
   Anjani putra Pavanasuta naama

   Ram's emissary, abode of matchless power, Anjani's son
   named "Son of the Wind."

9. **Mahaabeera birkama bajarangee,**
   Kumati nivaara sumati ke sangee

   Great hero, mighty as a thunderbolt, Remover of evil
   thoughts and companion to the good.

10. **Kanchana barana biraaja subesaa,**
    Kaanana kundala kunchita kesaa

    Golden-hued and splendidly adorned, With heavy
    earrings and curly locks.

11. Haatha bajra aura dvajaa biraajai,
    Kaandhe mooja janeu saajai

    *In your hands shine mace and banner, A sacred thread
    of munja grass adorns your shoulder.*

12. Shankara suvana Kesaree nandana,
    Teja prataapa mahaa jaga bandana

    *You are Shiva's son and Kesari's joy, Your glory is
    revealed throughout the world.*

13. Vidyaa vaana gunee ati chaatura,
    Raama kaaja karibe ko aatura

    *Supremely wise, virtuous and clever, You are ever intent
    on doing Ram's work.*

14. Prabhu charitra sunibe ko rasiyaa,
    Raama Lakshana Seetaa mana basiyaa

    *You delight in hearing of the Lord's deeds, Ram,
    Lakshman and Sita dwell in your heart.*

15. Sookshma roopa dhari Siyahin dikhaavaa,
    Bikata roopa dhari Lanka jaraavaa

    *Assuming tiny form you appeared to Sita, and in
    awesome guise you burned Lanka.*

16. Bheema roopa dhari asura sanghaare,
    Raamachandra ke kaaja sanvaare

    *Taking dreadful form you slaughtered demons and
    completed Lord Ram's mission.*

17. **Laaya sajeevana Lakhana jiyaaye,**
    Shree Raghubeera harashi ura laaye

    Bringing the magic herb, you revived Lakshman, and
    Ram embraced you with delight.

18. **Raghupati keenhee bahuta baraai,**
    tuma mama priya Bharatahi sama bhaai

    Greatly did the Raghu Lord praise you, "Brother, you're
    as dear to me as Bharati!"

19. **Sahasa badana tumharo jasa gaaven,**
    Asa kahi Shreepati kantha lagaaven

    "May the thousand-mouthed serpent sing your fame!" So
    saying, Shri's (Lakshmi's) Lord drew you to Himself.

20. **Sanakaadika Brahmaadi muneesaa,**
    Naarada Saarada sahita Aheesaa

    Sanak and the sages, Brahma, gods and great saints,
    Narada, Sarasvati and the King of serpents.

21. **Yama Kubera digapaala jahaante,**
    Kabi kobida kahi sake kahaante

    Yama, Kubera and the guardians of the four quadrants,
    Poets and scholars—none can express your glory.

22. **Tuma upakaara Sugreevahin keenhaa,**
    Raama milaaya raaja pada deenha

    You rendered great service to Sugriva, Presenting him to
    Ram, you give him kingship.

23. Tumharo mantra Vibheeshana maanaa,
    Lankeshvara bhaye saba jaga jaanaa

    *Vibhishana heeded your counsel and became Lord of
    Lanka, as all the world knows.*

24. Yuga sahasra jojana para bhaanu,
    Leelyo taahi madhura phala jaanu

    *Though the sun is thousands of miles away, You
    swallowed it, thinking it a sweet fruit.*

25. Prabhu mudrikaa meli mukha maaheen,
    Jaladhi laanghi gaye acharaja naaheen

    *Holding the Lord's ring in your mouth, it's no surprise
    you leapt over the ocean.*

26. Durgama kaaja jagata ke jete,
    Sugama anugraha tumhare tete

    *Every arduous task in this world becomes easy by your
    grace.*

27. Raama duaare tuma rakhavaare,
    Hota na aagyaa binu paisaare

    *You are the guardian of Ram's door; None enters
    without your leave.*

28. Saba sukha lahai tumhaaree sharanaa,
    Tuma rakshaka kaahu ko daranaa

    *Taking refuge in you one finds all delight; Those you
    protect know no fear.*

29. **Aapana teja samhaaru aapai,**
    Teenon loka haanka ten kaanpai

    You alone can withstand your own splendor; The three
    worlds tremble at your roar.

30. **Bhoota pisaacha nikata nahin aavai,**
    Mahaabeera jaba naama sunaavai

    Ghosts and goblins cannot come near, Great Hero, when
    your name is uttered.

31. **Naasai roga hare saba peeraa,**
    Japata nirantara Hanumata beeraa

    All disease and pain is eradicated, Brave Hanuman, by
    constant repetition of your name.

32. **Sankata tena Hanumaana churaavai,**
    Mana krama bachana dhyaana jo laavai

    Hanuman releases from affliction those who remember
    him in thought, word and deed.

33. **Saba para Raama tapaswee raajaa,**
    Tina ke kaaja sakala tuma saajaa

    Ram the ascetic reigns over all, but you carry out His
    every task.

34. **Aura Manoratha jo koee laave,**
    Soee amita jeevana phala paave

    One who comes to you with any yearning, Obtains the
    abundance of the Four Fruits of Life.

35. Chaaron yuga parataapa tumhaaraa,
    Hai parasidha jagata ujiyaaraa

    *Your splendor fills the four ages; Your glory is famed
    throughout the world.*

36. Saadhu santa ke tuma rakhavaara,
    Asura nikandana Raama dulaare

    *You are the guardian of saints and sages, the destroyer of
    demons, the darling of Ram.*

37. Ashta sidhi nau nidhi ke daataa,
    Asa bara deena Jaanakee Maataa

    *You grant the eight powers and nine treasures, By the
    boon you received from Mother Janaki (Sita).*

38. Raama rasaayana toomhare paasaa,
    Sadaa raho Raghupati ke daasaa

    *You hold the elixir of Ram's name and remain eternally
    his servant.*

39. Tumhare Bhajana Raama ko Paavai,
    Janama janama ke dukha bisaraavai

    *Singing your praise, one finds Ram and escapes the
    sorrows of countless lives.*

40. Anta kaala Raghubara pura jaeee,
    Jahaan janma Hari bhakta kahaaee

    *At death, one goes to Ram's own city or is born on earth
    as God's devotee.*

41. **Aura devataa chita na dharaee,**
    Hanumata se sarva sukha karaee

    Even if you give no thought to any other deity,
    Worshipping Hanuman, one gains all delight.

42. **Sankata katai mite saba peeraa,**
    Jo sumire Hanumata bala beeraa

    All affliction ceases, all pain is removed by remembering
    the mighty hero, Hanuman.

43. **Jai Jai Jai Hanumaana Gosaaee,**
    Kripaa karahu gurudeva kee naaee

    Victory, victory, victory to Lord Hanuman! Bestow your
    grace on me, as my Guru.

44. **Jo sata baara paata kara koeee,**
    Chootahi bandi mahaa sukha hoee

    Whoever recites this a hundred times is released from
    bondage and gains bliss.

45. **Jo yaha parai Hanumaana Chaleesa,**
    Hoya sidhi saakhee Gaureesaa

    One who reads this Hanuman Chalisa gains success as
    Gauri's Lord (Shiva) is witness.

46. **Tulaseedaasa sadaa Hari cheraa,**
    Keeje naata hridaya mahan deraa

    Says Tulsidas, Hari's constant servant, "Lord, make
    Your home in my heart."

47. Pawana tanaya sankata harana
    Mangala moorati roopa
    > *Son of the Wind, destroyer of sorrow, embodiment of blessings*

48. **Raama Lakhana Seetaa sahita,**
    Hridaya basahu sura bhoopa
    > *Dwell in my heart, King of Gods, together with Ram, Lakshman and Sita.*

49. **Mangala moorati Maruta nandan,**
    Sakala mangala moola nikandan
    > *Embodiment of welfare and auspiciousness, Son of the Wind, Source of All Blessings, Destroyer of All Limitation at the Root.*

Jai Bajrangbali Maharaj ki Jai![33]

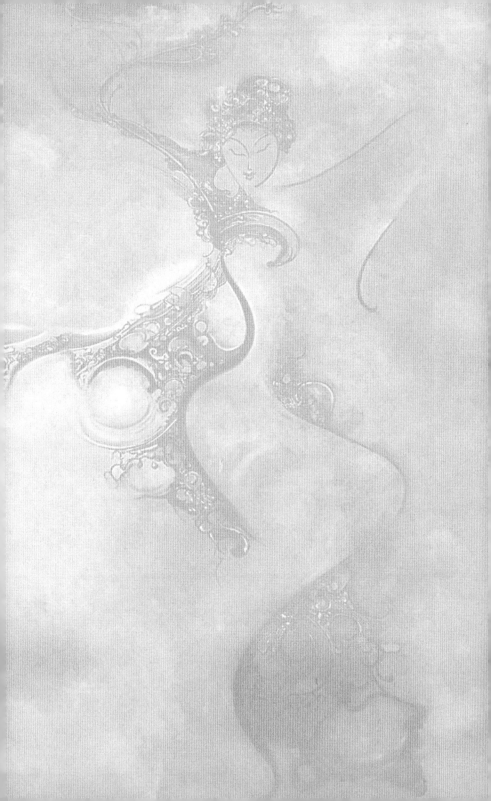

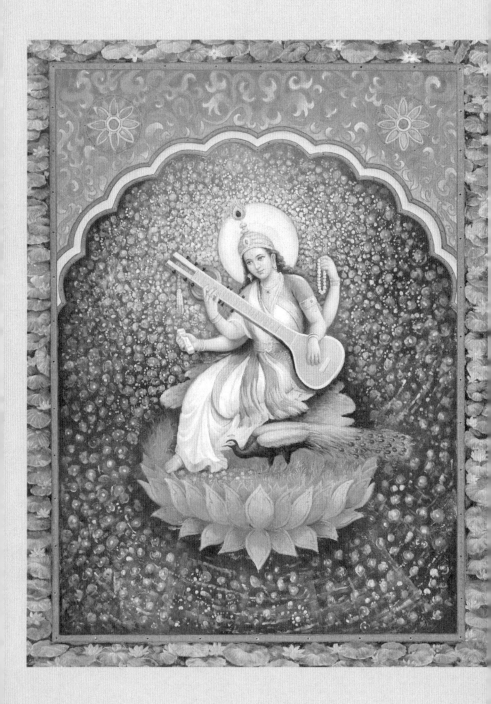

Chapter 16

Shakti Mantras

Mother dwells at the center of my being,
forever delightfully at play.
Whatever conditions of consciousness may arise,
I hear through them the music of her life-giving names,
Om Tara, Om Kali.

—Ramprasad Sen, trans. Lex Hixon

In the Tantric worldview, Shakti is the dynamic, Divine energy at play as all and everything. Sometimes referred to as the Divine Mother, this evolutionary energy is experienced as the grace-bestowing feminine principle that guides us from lifetime to lifetime. Taking a wondrous array of archetypal forms—Durga, Kali, Saraswati, and more—each with their own unique Divine qualities, this Shakti is also our own true life-force and identity. In fact, she embodies an all-encompassing vision of Oneness, as the ancient scripture the *Shakradi Stuti* reveals: "O Mother, this whole Universe is solely the movement of your Divine energy. Your form embodies the powers of all the gods." The yogic path of invoking and awakening to the Divine Mother is ultimately a journey of discovering our own true nature in Oneness with this supreme principle.

The Shakti mantras and chants in this section are powerful expressions of this Goddess wisdom. We can embrace these practices to cultivate greater depth and vibrancy of spiritual insight and experience, to dissolve difficulties and limitations in our lives that would obscure our highest manifestation, and to awaken to an embodied experience of our true Divine essence. The yogic path of Shakti represents the unifying embrace of the Divine dance of life—the *Lila*—affirming the living presence of the Divine in and as everyone and everything we experience.

The poems of Ramprasad Sen, an enlightened poet and devotee of Divine Mother wisdom, are like radiant windows into the living experience of this Shakti tradition. His ecstatic poems are love songs to Mother reality, offering us illuminating glimpses of our own Divine nature.

O human mind, while thinking and perceiving,
invoke instinctively the subtle sound *Om Kali*.
Why not ground your entire being in her living name
that dissolves all dangers arising
from without and from within?
How can you forget, even for an instant,
the innate cry *Ma! Ma! Ma!*
that resounds throughout the worlds?

✦ ✦ ✦

O mundane mind,
stop thinking in habitual patterns,
move beyond the structure of past, present, future,
leave your obsession with temporality.
Without care or regret, sing *Ma Tara, Ma Kali*.
Sail smoothly across the ocean of relativity.

＊ ＊ ＊

Overcome with fervent love, this poet pleads:
"O mind, how can you possibly forget the Goddess?
At the very center of your being
sing ceaselessly the name of Kali
and drink her deathless nectar.
Your life in the deceptive current of time
is coming to an end.
Soon you will know only Mother."

—*Ramprasad Sen*[34]

Shakti Mantras

The following mantras are best suited for japa mala practice. You can hear the pronunciation of the following mantras in the audio link below.

Shakti Mantras 1–4: GirishMusic.com/BookAudio

1. Om Shri Durgaayai Namah

The primary mantra of Durga, the Remover of Difficulties. This mantra is often used for internal and external protection as well as to bestow wisdom and strength.

2. Om Dum Durgaayai Namah

A mantra that invokes the energy of Durga, the Remover of Difficulties. This mantra can be used for protection against internal and external negative forces, and to bestow strength and wisdom. *The mantra can be translated as, "Salutations to Durga, the Divine Protectress," enhanced by Durga's seed-sound "Dum."*

3. Om Aim Hreem Kleem Chamundaayai Vicche Namah

This powerful mantra brings forth the experience of our true, higher nature by dissolving illusion. It can be chanted for purification, protection, and to dissolve negativities. It is said to bestow self-confidence, self-esteem, and power, particularly for women. The mantra can be translated as, "Salutations to Chamundi (a fierce aspect of Shakti) who destroys negativity."

4. Om Aim Saraswatyai Namah

A mantra to attune to the energy of Saraswati, bringing forth her creative blossoming in music, creativity and the arts, spiritual knowledge, and Divine speech. The mantra can be translated as, "Salutations to Saraswati, the one who leads to the essence of self-knowledge."[35]

Saraswati Maha Vidya Mantra

Saraswati Maha Vidya Mantra: GirishMusic.com/BookAudio

Aim Hreem Shreem Kleem
Sauh Kleem Hreem Aim
Bloom Streem Neelatari Saraswati
Draam Dreem Kleem Bloom

Sah Aim Hreem Shreem
Kleem Sauh Sauh Hreem Swaha

> The Saraswati Maha Vidya *is a powerful mantra known as "The Queen of Knowledge." Chanting this mantra can bring great spiritual knowledge through the grace of Saraswati, the Goddess of Divine Speech. Since this mantra is a series of bija mantras or seed-sounds, it is not really translatable.*

Devi Suktam Hymn

The *Devi Suktam* is an ancient and powerful hymn, invoking and revealing the many Divine qualities of Shakti. This chant originally appears in the oldest known Hindu scripture, the *Rig Veda*. It is chanted by yogis to remove the obscuring identification with "I" and "mine," allowing our true Divine nature to shine forth. You'll find the recorded version of this text chant in the audio link.

Devi Suktam: GirishMusic.com/BookAudio

1. **Namo Devyai Mahaadevyai**
   Shivaayai Satatam Namah
   Namah Prakrityai Bhadraayai
   Niyataah Pranataah Sma Taam

   > *We bow to the Goddess, to the Great Goddess, to the Energy of Infinite Goodness at all times we bow. We bow to Nature, to the Excellent One, with discipline we have bowed down.*

2. Raudraayai Namo Nityaayai
   Gauryai Dhaatryai Namo Namah
   Jyotsnaayai Chenduroopinyai
   Suhkaayai Satatam Namah

   > To the Reliever of Sufferings we bow, to the Eternal, to
   > the Embodiment of Rays of Light, to the Creatress, to
   > She Who Manifests Light, to the form of Devotion, to
   > Happiness continually we bow.

3. Kalyaanyai Pranataam Vriddhyai
   Siddhyai Kurmo Namo Namah
   Nairrityai Bhoobhritaam Lakshmyai
   Sharvaanyai Te Namo Namah

   > To the Welfare of those who bow, we bow; to Change, to
   > Perfection, to Dissolution, to the Wealth that sustains the
   > earth, to the Wife of Consciousness, to You, we bow, we bow.

4. Durgaayai Durgapaaraayai
   Saaraayai Sarvakaarinyai
   Khyaatyai Tathaiva Krishnaayai
   Dhoomraayai Satatam Namah

   > To She Who Removes Difficulties, to She Who Removes
   > Beyond All Difficulties, to the Essence, to the Cause
   > of All; to Perception, and to the Doer of All, to the
   > Unknowable One, continually we bow.

5. Atisaumyaati Raudraayai
   Nataastasyai Namo Namah
   Namo Jagat Pratishtaayai
   Devyai Krityai Namo Namah

*To the extremely beautiful and to the extremely fierce, we
bow to Her, we bow, we bow. We bow to the Establisher
of the Perceivable Universe, to the Goddess, to All
Action, we bow, we bow.*

**6. Yaa Devi Sarva Bhooteshu Vishnu Maayeti Shabditaa
Namastasyai Namastasyai Namastasyai Namo Namah**

*To the Divine Goddess in all existence who is addressed
as the Perceivable Form of the Consciousness Which
Pervades All, we bow to Her; we bow to Her, we bow to
Her, continually we bow, we bow.*

**7. Yaa Devi Sarva Bhooteshu Chetanetyabhi Dheeyate
Namastasyai Namastasyai Namastasyai Namo Namah**

*To the Divine Goddess in all existence who resides
all throughout Consciousness and is known by the
reflections of mind, we bow to Her; we bow to Her, we
bow to Her, continually we bow, we bow.*

**8. Yaa Devi Sarva Bhooteshu Buddhiroopena Samsthitaa
Namastasyai Namastasyai Namastasyai Namo Namah**

*To the Divine Goddess who resides in all existence in the
form of Intelligence, we bow to Her; we bow to Her, we
bow to Her, continually we bow, we bow.*

**9. Yaa Devi Sarva Bhooteshu Nidraaroopena Samsthitaa
Namastasyai Namastasyai Namastasyai Namo Namah**

*To the Divine Goddess who resides in all existence in the
form of Sleep, we bow to Her; we bow to Her, we bow to
Her, continually we bow, we bow.*

10. Yaa Devi Sarva Bhooteshu Kshudhaaroopena Samsthitaa
Namastasyai Namastasyai Namastasyai Namo Namah
*To the Divine Goddess who resides in all existence in the
form of Hunger, we bow to Her; we bow to Her, we bow
to Her, continually we bow, we bow.*

11. Yaa Devi Sarva Bhooteshu Chaayaaroopena Samsthitaa
Namastasyai Namastasyai Namastasyai Namo Namah
*To the Divine Goddess who resides in all existence in the
form of Appearance, we bow to Her; we bow to Her, we
bow to Her, continually we bow, we bow.*

12. Yaa Devi Sarva Bhooteshu Shaktiroopena Samsthitaa
Namastasyai Namastasyai Namastasyai Namo Namah
*To the Divine Goddess who resides in all existence in the
form of Energy, we bow to Her; we bow to Her, we bow
to Her, continually we bow, we bow.*

13. Yaa Devi Sarva Bhooteshu Trishnaaroopena Samsthitaa
Namastasyai Namastasyai Namastasyai Namo Namah
*To the Divine Goddess who resides in all existence in the
form of Desire, we bow to Her; we bow to Her, we bow
to Her, continually we bow, we bow.*

14. Yaa Devi Sarva Bhooteshu Kshaantiroopena Samsthitaa
Namastasyai Namastasyai Namastasyai Namo Namah
*To the Divine Goddess who resides in all existence in the
form of Patient Forgiveness, we bow to Her; we bow to
Her, we bow to Her, continually we bow, we bow.*

15. **Yaa Devi Sarva Bhooteshu Jaatiroopena Samsthitaa Namastasyai Namastasyai Namastasyai Namo Namah**

    To the Divine Goddess who resides in all existence in the form of All Living Beings, we bow to Her; we bow to Her, we bow to Her, continually we bow, we bow.

16. **Yaa Devi Sarva Bhooteshu Lajjaaroopena Samsthitaa Namastasyai Namastasyai Namastasyai Namo Namah**

    To the Divine Goddess who resides in all existence in the form of Humility, we bow to Her; we bow to Her, we bow to Her, continually we bow, we bow.

17. **Yaa Devi Sarva Bhooteshu Shaantiroopena Samsthitaa Namastasyai Namastasyai Namastasyai Namo Namah**

    To the Divine Goddess who resides in all existence in the form of Peace, we bow to Her; we bow to Her, we bow to Her, continually we bow, we bow.

18. **Yaa Devi Sarva Bhooteshu Shraddhaaroopena Samsthitaa Namastasyai Namastasyai Namastasyai Namo Namah**

    To the Divine Goddess who resides in all existence in the form of Faith, we bow to Her; we bow to Her, we bow to Her, continually we bow, we bow.

19. **Yaa Devi Sarva Bhooteshu Kaantiroopena Samsthitaa Namastasyai Namastasyai Namastasyai Namo Namah**

    To the Divine Goddess who resides in all existence in the form of Beauty Enhanced by Love, we bow to Her; we bow to Her, we bow to Her, continually we bow, we bow.

**20. Yaa Devi Sarva Bhooteshu Lakshmeeroopena Samsthitaa
Namastasyai Namastasyai Namastasyai Namo Namah**
*To the Divine Goddess who resides in all existence in the
form of True Wealth, we bow to Her; we bow to Her, we
bow to Her, continually we bow, we bow.*

**21. Yaa Devi Sarva Bhooteshu Vrittiroopena Samsthitaa
Namastasyai Namastasyai Namastasyai Namo Namah**
*To the Divine Goddess who resides in all existence in the
form of Activity, we bow to Her; we bow to Her, we bow
to Her, continually we bow, we bow.*

**22. Yaa Devi Sarva Bhooteshu Smritiroopena Samsthitaa
Namastasyai Namastasyai Namastasyai Namo Namah**
*To the Divine Goddess who resides in all existence in the
form of Recollection, we bow to Her; we bow to Her, we
bow to Her, continually we bow, we bow.*

**23. Yaa Devi Sarva Bhooteshu Dayaaroopena Samsthitaa
Namastasyai Namastasyai Namastasyai Namo Namah**
*To the Divine Goddess who resides in all existence in the
form of Compassion, we bow to Her; we bow to Her, we
bow to Her, continually we bow, we bow.*

**24. Yaa Devi Sarva Bhooteshu Tushtiroopena Samsthitaa
Namastasyai Namastasyai Namastasyai Namo Namah**
*To the Divine Goddess who resides in all existence in the
form of Satisfaction, we bow to Her; we bow to Her, we
bow to Her, continually we bow, we bow.*

25. Yaa Devi Sarva Bhooteshu Maatriroopena Samsthitaa
Namastasyai Namastasyai Namastasyai Namo Namah
*To the Divine Goddess who resides in all existence in the
form of Mother, we bow to Her; we bow to Her, we bow
to Her, continually we bow, we bow.*

26. Yaa Devi Sarva Bhooteshu Bhraantiroopena Samsthitaa
Namastasyai Namastasyai Namastasyai Namo Namah
*To the Divine Goddess who resides in all existence in the
form of Confusion, we bow to Her; we bow to Her, we
bow to Her, continually we bow, we bow.*

27. Indriyaanaam-adhishthaatri
Bhootaanaam Chaakileshu Yaa
Bhooteshu Satatam Tasyai
Vyaaptidevyai Namo Namah
*Presiding over the senses of all beings and pervading
all existence, to the Omnipresent Goddess who
individualizes creation we bow, we bow.*

28. Chitiroopena Yaa Kritsna-
Metad Vyaapya Sthitaa Jagat
Namastasyai Namastasyai
Namastasyai Namo Namah
*In the form of Consciousness, She distinguishes the individual
phenomena of the perceivable Universe. We bow to Her, we
bow to Her, we bow to Her; continually we bow, we bow.*

Om Shanti Shanti Shanti
Om Peace, Peace, Peace[36]

Shri Devi Ashtottara Chant:
108 Names of the Divine Mother

The *Shri Devi Ashtottara* is an inspiring and empowering collection of 108 names of the Goddess, hand-selected by Shankaracharya Swami of the MahaShakti Yoga lineage. This is a profoundly powerful invocation of Shakti, one which is quite easy to chant because of its simple, repetitive melody. You'll find the recorded version of this text chant in the audio link.

Shri Devi Ashtottara: GirishMusic.com/BookAudio

1. **Om Hreem Durgaayai Namah**
   Salutations to She who Is Unattainable
2. **Om Lakshmyai Namah**
   Is Good Fortune
3. **Om Lajjaayai Namah**
   Is Modesty
4. **Om Shraddhaayai Namah**
   Is Faith
5. **Om Pushtyai Namah**
   Is Nourishing
6. **Om Svadhaayai Namah**
   Is the Praise of Ancestors
7. **Om Mahaaraatyai Namah**
   Is the Stillness into which All Forms Dissolve
8. **Om Mahaamaayaayai Namah**
   Is the Great Veiling Power

9. **Om Medhaayai Namah**
   Is Intelligence
10. **Om Maatre Namah**
   Is the Divine Mother
11. **Om Sarasvatyai Namah**
   Is Knowledge
12. **Om Shivaayai Namah**
   Is the Energy of Shiva
13. **Om Shashidharaayai Namah**
   Bears the Moon of Life's Nectar
14. **Om Shaantaayai Namah**
   Is Peace
15. **Om Shaambhavyai Namah**
   Is Sacred to Shiva
16. **Om Buddhidaayinyai Namah**
   Grants Intelligence
17. **Om Taamasyai Namah**
   Is the Darkness of the Void
18. **Om Niyataayai Namah**
   Restrains
19. **Om Naaryai Namah**
   Is the Universal Woman
20. **Om Naaraayanyai Namah**
   Is Unlimited Consciousness
21. **Om Kaalyai Namah**
   Is Beyond Time
22. **Om Kalaayai Namah**
   Is the Single Part
23. **Om Brahmyai Namah**
   Is Creative Energy

24. **Om Bhagavatyai Namah**
    Is Adorable
25. **Om Vanyai Namah**
    Is Abundance
26. **Om Shaaradaayai Namah**
    Is Supreme Knowledge
27. **Om Hamsavaahinyai Namah**
    Rides the Swan of Vital Breath
28. **Om Trishoolinyai Namah**
    Carries the Trident of Nature's Three Qualities
29. **Om Trinetraayai Namah**
    Has Three Eyes
30. **Om Ishaayai Namah**
    Is the Supreme Spirit
31. **Om Traayai Namah**
    Protects
32. **Om Shubhaayai Namah**
    Is Shining
33. **Om Satyaayai Namah**
    Is Truth
34. **Om Kaushikyai Namah**
    Springs from Parvati's Sheath
35. **Om Gauryai Namah**
    Is Sublime
36. **Om Karaalyai Namah**
    Is Formidable
37. **Om Maalinyai Namah**
    Is Garlanded
38. **Om Madhyai Namah**
    Is the Middle

39. **Om Maheshvaryai Namah**
    Is Supreme, Without Attributes
40. **Om Maheshagnyai Namah**
    Is the Great Goddess of Fire
41. **Om Madhuvrataayai Namah**
    Is Sweetness
42. **Om Mahaashaktyai Namah**
    Is Supreme Power
43. **Om Bhaaratyai Namah**
    Is Speech
44. **Om Bhuvaneshvaryai Namah**
    Is the Mother of the Worlds
45. **Om Pitaayai Namah**
    Is the Father
46. **Om Kaumaaryai Namah**
    Is Pure
47. **Om Raajanyai Namah**
    Is Royal
48. **Om Raadhinyai Namah**
    Is Prosperity
49. **Om Raktaayai Namah**
    Is Charming
50. **Om Chaamundaayai Namah**
    Destroys Selfish Passion and Meanness
51. **Om Paarvatyai Namah**
    Is the Mountain Daughter
52. **Om Prabhaayai Namah**
    Is Luminous
53. **Om Nishumbapraanahaarinyai Namah**
    Disposes of Malice

54. **Om Kanyaayai Namah**
    Is the Girl
55. **Om Raktabeejanipaatinyai Namah**
    Destroys the Seeds of Desire
56. **Om Sahasravadanaayai Namah**
    Has Endless Forms
57. **Om Sandhyaayai Namah**
    Is the Time of Worship
58. **Om Saakshinyai Namah**
    Is the Witness
59. **Om Shankaryai Namah**
    Is Auspicious
60. **Om Dyutaayai Namah**
    Is Splendor
61. **Om Bhargavyai Namah**
    Is Effulgence
62. **Om Vaarunyai Namah**
    Is the Mother of Water
63. **Om Vidyaayai Namah**
    Is All Knowledge
64. **Om Dhaaraayai Namah**
    Supports All
65. **Om Gaayatryai Namah**
    Is the Mother of Hymns
66. **Om Gaayakshyai Namah**
    Sings
67. **Om Gangaayai Namah**
    Is Sacred Water
68. **Om Chandeekaayai Namah**
    Is Fierce

69. **Om Gitaganasvaraayai Namah**
    Is the Praises Sung
70. **Om Chandomayaayai Namah**
    Is the Meter of Sacred Hymns
71. **Om Mahyai Namah**
    Is the Greatest
72. **Om Chaayaayai Namah**
    Is Reflection
73. **Om Chandanpriyaayai Namah**
    Loves Sandalwood
74. **Om Jananyai Namah**
    Is All Existence
75. **Om Yoginyai Namah**
    Is the Possessor of Yoga
76. **Om Shambhovyai Namah**
    Is the Source of All Happiness
77. **Om Vallaryai Namah**
    Is a Cluster of Blossoms
78. **Om Vallabhaayai Namah**
    Is Most Beloved
79. **Om Haritakshyai Namah**
    Gives Form to Vishnu
80. **Om Hariharapriyaayai Namah**
    Is the Beloved of Shiva and Vishnu
81. **Om Bhootyai Namah**
    Is the Mother of All That Is
82. **Om Tripurasundaaryai Namah**
    Is the Beauty Pervading the Spheres
83. **Om Varahastaayai Namah**
    Grants Blessings

84. **Om Ambikaayai Namah**
   Is Venerable

85. **Om Sarvasiddhaayai Namah**
   Is Perfection in Everything

86. **Om Saravidyaayai Namah**
   Is the Water of Knowledge

87. **Om Dinaayai Namah**
   Creates the Day

88. **Om Dootaayai Namah**
   Is the Emissary of Perfection

89. **Om Devyai Namah**
   Is the Supreme Goddess

90. **Om Duhkha Haraayai Namah**
   Takes Away Pain

91. **Om Dinasiddhaayai Namah**
   Makes the Day Perfect

92. **Om Digambaryai Namah**
   Is Clothed in Space

93. **Om Devakanyaayai Namah**
   Is the Daughter of the Gods

94. **Om Devasiddhaayai Namah**
   Is the Perfection of the Gods

95. **Om Devapoojaayai Namah**
   Is Worshipped by the Gods

96. **Om Devadhanaayai Namah**
   Is the Wealth of the Gods

97. **Om Devakaamaayai Namah**
   Is the Gods' Desire

98. **Om Dayaayai Namah**
   Is Compassionate

99. **Om Daatriyai Namah**
    Gives
100. **Om Dakshakanaayai Namah**
    Is the Most Able Daughter
101. **Om Dakshamaatre Namah**
    Is the Most Able Mother
102. **Om Devadevapriyaayai Namah**
    Is the Beloved of the Gods
103. **Om Nitya Muktaayai Namah**
    Is Eternally Liberated
104. **Om Nitya Shaantaayai Namah**
    Is Eternally Peaceful
105. **Om Nirvikalpaayai Namah**
    Is Beyond Thought
106. **Om Yoga Siddhaayai Namah**
    Is the Perfection of Union
107. **Om Parameshvaryai Namah**
    Is the Supreme Being
108. **Om Aadyaayai Namah**
    Is Primordial[37]

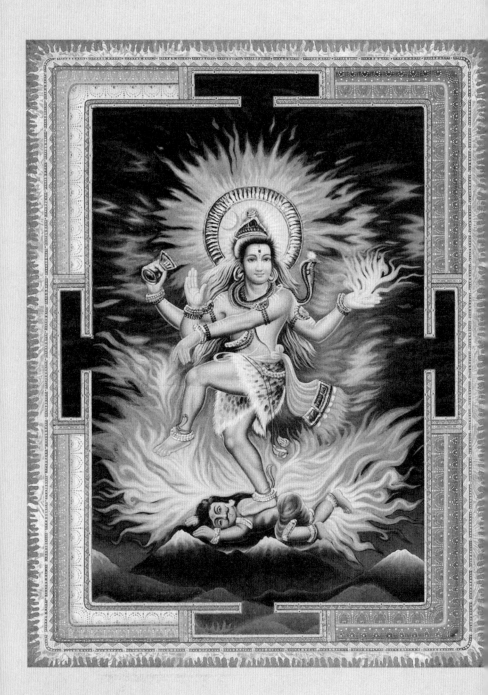

Chapter 17

Shiva Mantras

Shiva is universally recognized as the Deity most associated with the path of yoga. He is known as the God of Wisdom, the Destroyer of Ignorance, and the Bestower of Joy. His name in Sanskrit literally means "the good one" or "the auspicious one." He exists both as the Divine archetype of pure wisdom beyond any trace of illusion as well as the embodiment of the original yogi, meditating in the exalted, snowy peaks of Mount Kailash in the Himalayas. Shiva is also the Divine healer, burning away the subtle seeds of karma that bring about physical, emotional, or psychological suffering, awakening a restorative healing force within us to bring longevity, vitality, well-being, and peace.

Shiva's iconography has been present for thousands of years in one form or another in spiritual and religious traditions not only in India, but in various cultures around the world. Some scholars trace the origins of Shiva back to a pre-Vedic people known as the Dravidians, who came to the Indian subcontinent from the eastern Mediterranean sometime around 7000 BC. In the ancient texts of India's *Vedas*, Shiva was synonymous with Rudra, the

Destroyer of Sorrow. In the *Yajur Veda*, Shiva is described as the inner self within all beings:

> *He is the Shining One, hidden in all beings,*
> *their inmost soul who is in all.*
> *He watches the works of creation, lives*
> *in all things, watches all things.*
> *He is pure consciousness, beyond the*
> *three conditions of nature.*

The great Indian saint and scholar Adi Shankaracharya described Shiva as "the One who purifies everyone by the very utterance of His name." He embodies a transcendent reality beyond the mind and rational thought, as the *Sama Veda* says:

> *There the eye goes not, nor words, nor mind. We know not. We*
> *cannot understand how He can be explained. He is above the*
> *known, and He is above the unknown.*

Whereas the path of Shakti is one of seeing and embracing the Divine in and as the world, the path of Shiva is one of transcendence, discriminating the unreal from the real—known through the aphorism "*Neti, neti,*" "Not this, not this." Once the illusion has been burned away through the gaze of Shiva's wisdom, we can glimpse the realization described in Adi Shankaracharya's *Nirvanashatkam*:

> *I am free from thoughts, and I have no form. I am all-pervading,*
> *beyond the senses, everywhere. I am unchanging and know*
> *neither liberation nor bondage. I am indeed, That eternal*
> *knowing and bliss, Shiva, love and pure consciousness.*

As you chant the sacred sounds and mantras of Shiva, allow your awareness to dwell in the Vishuddha (throat), Ajna (third eye), or Sahasrara (crown) chakra centers, opening yourself to the subtle inner light of wisdom. Let your awareness gradually ascend beyond ordinary identification with body and mind, into the blissful experience of pure being and consciousness.

Shiva Mantras

The following mantras are best suited for japa mala practice. You can hear the pronunciation of the following mantras in the audio link below.

Shiva Mantras 1–3: GirishMusic.com/BookAudio

1. Om Namah Shivaya

A mantra for transformation, awakening, and healing. It means, "I honor the inner Self, Shiva, the light of consciousness within me." This mantra contains the five primal sounds of the elements ("Na" = earth, "Ma" = water, "Shi" = fire, "Va" = air, and "Ya" = ether). Thus, as we chant the sounds of this mantra we are ascending vibrationally from an earthly, physically oriented awareness to a subtler, higher state of consciousness.

2. Om Hreem Haum Namah Shivaya

This is a powerful Shiva mantra, enhanced with the seed-sounds of "Hreem" (embodying Shakti's energy as the "lightning bolt" which allows us to see through

illusion and glimpse our true higher nature) and
"Haum" (embodying Shiva's energy as pure awakened
consciousness).

3. **Om Shreem Kleem Namah Shivaya**
   A mantra for abundant manifestation that connects and
   attunes us to the elements of creation. This mantra can
   be translated as, "Om and salutations to Shiva, He who
   embraces all consciousness," enhanced with the seed-
   sounds "Shreem" for Lakshmi's abundance and "Kleem"
   for attraction.[38]

Mahamrityunjaya Mantra

With this mantra one is able to conquer all one's
enemies (anger, hatred, jealousy, and greed). It is
the source of longevity, health, and well-being . . .
Assuming different forms and shapes, the power
of this light, the Mrityunjaya mantra pervades the
whole universe. It is the source of all protection,
physical, mental, and spiritual.

—*NETRA TANTRA*,
TRANS. PANDIT RAJMANI TIGUNAIT, PHD

The great *Mahamrityunjaya* mantra stands alongside the *Gayatri*
mantra as one of the most revered sacred chants for meditation
and spiritual awakening. It is known as Shiva's *Maha Moksha*
mantra, or "Great Liberation" mantra, and is said to impart the

experience of our eternal Divine nature. While the *Mahamrityunjaya* is sometimes used as a means of protection against death, calamity, or disease, the mantra also has renowned restorative and healing properties and is said to bestow longevity and vitality. In fact, some Ayurvedic physicians recommend chanting the *Mahamrityunjaya* to enhance the healing effects of medicines they prescribe.

The *Mahamrityunjaya* may be chanted out loud in the style recorded in the audio link, or done as part of a japa mala practice.

Mahamrityunjaya Mantra: GirishMusic.com/BookAudio

1. **Mahamrityunjaya Mantra**
   Om Trayambakam Yajaamahae
   Sugandhim Pushti Vardhanam
   Urvaarukamiva Bandhanaan
   Mrityor Muksheeya Maamritaat

   I surrender myself to the Divine Being (Shiva) who
   embodies the power of will, the power of knowledge,
   and the power of action. I pray to the Divine Being who
   manifests in the form of fragrance in the flower of life
   and is the eternal nourisher of the plant of life. Like a
   skillful gardener, may the Lord of Life disentangle me
   from the binding forces of my physical, psychological,
   and spiritual foes. May the lord of Immortality residing
   within me, free me from death, decay and sickness and
   unite me with immortality.

Nirvanashatkam

The *Nirvanashatkam*, sometimes called the "Song of the Self," is a text chant that embodies the bliss and freedom of self-realization, expressed in six luminous verses by the great sage Adi Shankaracharya. As a boy, Shankaracharya was said to be wandering in the Himalayas in search of a worthy spiritual guide, when he came upon the sage Gaudapada, who asked him, "Who are you?" The young Shankaracharya's enlightened reply has been a source of inspiration for seekers of truth since the eighth century.

Each of the six verses of this wisdom chant gradually dissolves every illusory limitation within and without, until all that remains is Shiva—our true nature as pure being, consciousness, and bliss. You'll find the recorded version of this text chant in the audio link.

Nirvanashatkam: GirishMusic.com/BookAudio

1. **Mano Buddhyahankaara Chittaani Naaham**
   Na Cha Shrotra Jihve Na Cha Ghraananetre
   Na Cha Vyomabhoomir Na Tejo Na Vaajuh
   Chidaanandaroopah Shivo'ham Shivo'ham

   I am not mind, nor intellect, nor ego, nor the reflections of inner self (chitta). I am not the five senses. I am beyond that. I am not the ether, nor the earth, nor the fire, nor the water, nor the wind (the five elements). I am indeed, That eternal knowing and bliss, Shiva, love and pure consciousness.

2. **Na Cha Praanasangyo Na Vai Panchavaayu**
   Na Vaa Saptadhaaturna Vaa Panchakoshah

Na Vaak Paanipaadau Na Chopasthapaayoo
Chidaanandaroopah Shivo'ham Shivo'ham

> *I am neither the life force nor the five kinds of vital air.
> I am neither the seven constituents of the body nor its
> five sheaths. I am not the organs of speech, movement,
> elimination or procreation. I am indeed, That eternal
> knowing and bliss, Shiva, love and pure consciousness.*

3. Na Me Dvesharaagau Na Me Lobhamohau
Mado Naiva Me Naiva Maatsaryahaavah
Na Dharmo Na Chaartho Na Kaamo Na Mokshah
Chidaanandaroopah Shivo'ham Shivo'ham

> *I am free from attraction and aversion, greed and
> delusion. I have neither pride nor envy, nor any sense of
> righteousness or success. No desire remains, not even for
> liberation. I am indeed, That eternal knowing and bliss,
> Shiva, love and pure consciousness.*

4. Na Punyam Na Paapam Na Saukhyam Na Duhkham
Na Mantro Na Teertham Na Vedaa na Yajnaah
Aham Bhojanam Naiva Bhojyam Na Bhoktaa
Chidaanandaroopah Shivo'ham Shivo'ham

> *I am neither right nor wrong action, pleasure nor pain.
> I am not the mantra, the holy site, the Vedas or the
> sacrifice. I am not enjoyment, the object of enjoyment or
> the one who enjoys. I am indeed, That eternal knowing
> and bliss, Shiva, love and pure consciousness.*

5. Na Me Mrityushankaa Na Me Jaatibhedah
Pitaa Naiva Me Naiva Maataa Na Janma
Na Bandhur Na Mitram Gurur Naiva Shishyah

Chidaanandaroopah Shivo'ham Shivo'ham

> *I have no fear of death. I know no distinction between myself and others. I have neither father nor mother, and I have never been born. I have neither brother nor friend, neither teacher nor student. I am indeed, That eternal knowing and bliss, Shiva, love and pure consciousness.*

6. **Aham Nirvikalpo Niraakaararoopo**
   Vibhurvyaapya Sarvatra Sarvendriyaanaam
   Sadaa Me Samatvam Na Muktir Na Bandhah
   Chidaanandaroopah Shivo'ham Shivo'ham

> *I am free from thoughts, and I have no form. I am all-pervading, beyond the senses, everywhere. I am unchanging and know neither liberation nor bondage. I am indeed, That eternal knowing and bliss, Shiva, love and pure consciousness.*[39]

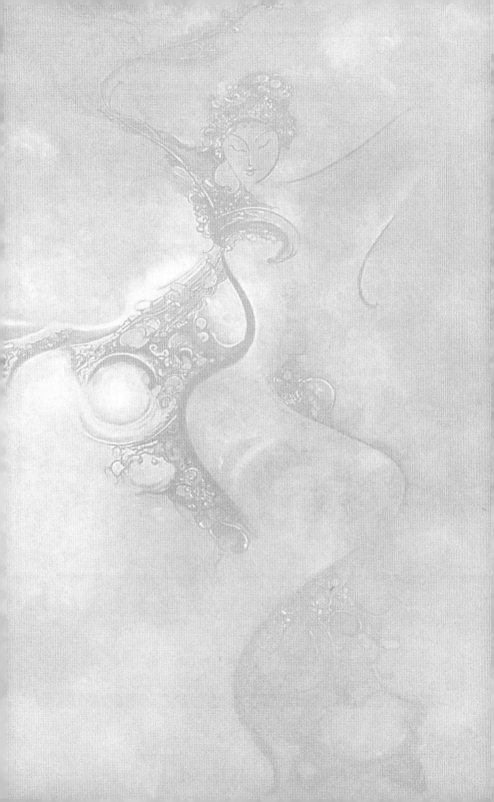

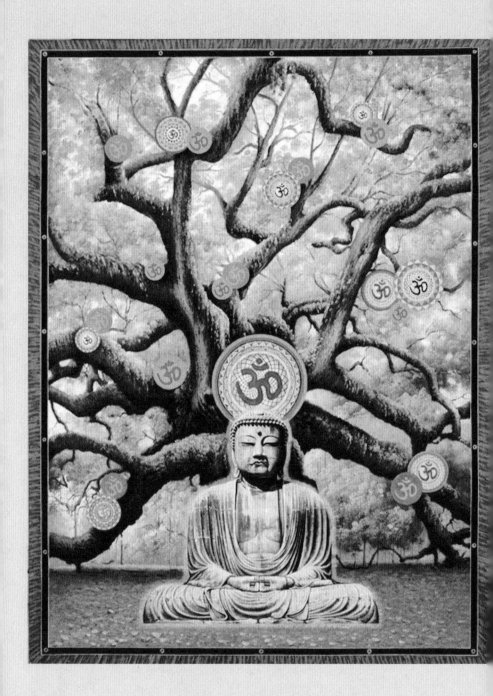

Chapter 18

Mantras for Love, Peace, and Wisdom

The following mantras are best suited for japa mala practice. You can hear the pronunciation of the following mantras in the audio link below.

Love, Peace, and Wisdom Mantras 1–4: GirishMusic.com/BookAudio

1. **Shante Prashante Sarva Bhaya Upashaya-Mani Svaha**

   A mantra for releasing fear. This chant invokes supreme peace by releasing fear back to its source in the universal mind. The energy is then purified and returned to us in usable, productive form.

2. **Aham Prema**

   A beautiful mantra to invoke the living energy of the highest Love within our hearts and lives, infusing every relationship and every situation we encounter. We are the embodiment of Love. This is a Love rooted in the spiritual experience of Oneness, compassion, and healing. The mantra can be translated to mean, "I am Divine Love."

3. Lokaah Samasthaah Sukhino Bhavantu

A mantra to express loving-kindness to all living beings, and to affirm our Unity with all existence. The mantra can be translated as, "May all beings, everywhere, be happy and free."

4. Sat Chid Ekam Brahma

A powerful mantra to begin or accelerate the process of accumulating true knowledge and wisdom. Swami Satyananda Saraswati translates it to mean, "Om. True Existence, Infinite Consciousness, One Supreme Divinity. I am one with God!" Thomas Ashley-Farrand writes that through chanting this mantra the secrets of the Universe reveal themselves to you.[40]

The Gayatri Mantra

The great *Gayatri* is a mantra of infinite spiritual energy, and is said to contain the essence of all mantras. Sometimes called "The Song of the Sun," this mantra is an ancient invocation of the Light within us and within everything. It is a deep prayer for spiritual liberation, both for ourselves and all living beings.

As one of the few mantras that is common to both Hinduism and Buddhism, the *Gayatri* is considered to be spiritual Light itself in the form of sound. Chanting this mantra illumines the mind and the intellect, awakening us to the experience of our Divine nature.

It may be chanted as part of a japa mala practice or chanted out loud. You'll find the recorded version of this mantra in the audio link.

Gayatri Mantra: GirishMusic.com/BookAudio

Gayatri Mantra

Om Bhur Bhuvah Svaha
Tat Savitur Varenyam
Bhargo Devasya Dheemahi
Dhiyo Yo Nah Prachodayaat

> *Let us meditate on the effulgent, eternal consciousness;*
> *that unseen force with no beginning and no ending,*
> *which has created the entire Universe. Absolute*
> *existence, consciousness, bliss, creation, and truth, who*
> *appears through transcendental light, illuminate our*
> *understanding. We meditate on that light. May all*
> *beings perceive the all-pervading brilliance of enlightened*
> *awareness.*

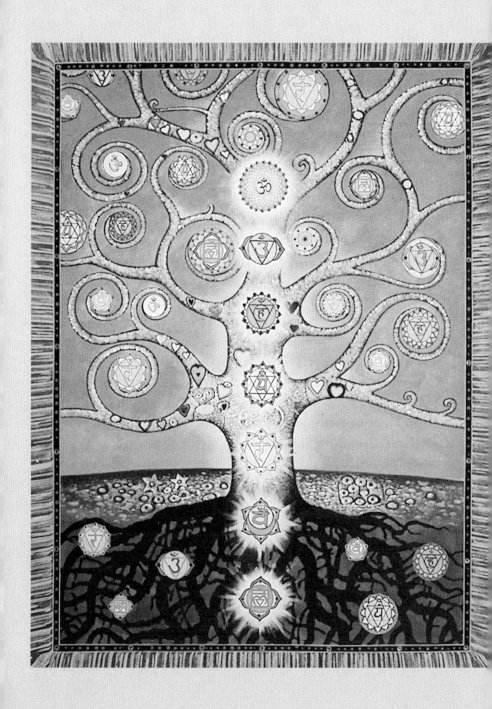

Conclusion:
40-Day Anusthan Practice

Whatever you ask for in prayer, believe that
you have received it, and it will be yours.

—Jesus

One year ago, when I first embarked on the journey of writing this book, I found myself filled with two clearly competing sets of emotions. Part of me felt overjoyed and honored to be called upon like this to share my experiences in the world of mantra. However, in stark opposition to this feeling of exhilaration, I would sometimes find myself overcome with self-doubt and even a sense of dread. That's when the inner critic would chime in with his unhelpful opinions, *You've never written a book before! How in the world do you think you're going to pull this off??*

Seeing that these old belief patterns (*samskaras*) were creating internal obstacles for my writing process, I decided to employ the most potent transformational tool that I know of: mantra practice. As an investment in my own personal growth and self-care, as well as a demonstration that I might share here on the pages of this book, I began a 40-day anusthan (period of unbroken practice) of a powerful Saraswati mantra. The Sanskrit roots of

239

this word *anusthan* show us the real meaning behind this powerful practice. The first root, *anu*, means "firm" or "direct," while the second root, *sthaana*, can be translated as "abode," "fortress," and "continuance in the same state." When we embrace the powerful practice of a 40-day anusthan, we immerse ourselves each day in the direct, embodied experience of our highest intentions, allowing the energies of those intentions to abide in us more and more until they become our living reality.

Considering the monumental undertaking I was about to embark upon, I wanted to choose a mantra that was appropriately epic in its energetic and transformative powers. After searching about through all of the Saraswati mantras I'd learned over the years, I felt a deep calling and connection to one in particular that I had never actually chanted before: the *Maha Vidya*, the "Queen of Knowledge" mantra (see Chapter 16).

As I've mentioned elsewhere, I'm not very rule-oriented when it comes to choosing a mantra. In my experience, it matters far less what one scripture or another says a mantra is supposed to be used for than it does what mantra we truly feel drawn to in our heart of hearts. And, for me, the *Maha Vidya* was that mantra. It felt to me like the right energetic ally to support me in fulfilling my intention of completing this book with the highest grace, wisdom, love, and joy possible.

As luck would have it, the full moon was coming up just a day after settling on my choice for which mantra to use. This seemed like an auspicious time to begin my journey into the presence and energy of Saraswati. So, that very next day, I began the 40-day practice.

In the Stream of Saraswati's Creative Flow

During the first few days of the practice, there was a clear process of acclimation to the sounds and energies of this very powerful and rather complicated mantra happening within me. I found myself stumbling over the new, unfamiliar sounds and having to follow along with a printed version of the mantra to remember how it went. This is a common experience, especially when we're new to a particular chant or to mantra in general. It's useful to be aware that for many of us in those first days of practice we may feel as if things haven't quite "clicked" yet. We may have the sense that we're too busy getting used to the sounds of a new mantra—how it goes—to be able to really notice its energetic qualities at all. But, rest assured, even from that very first recitation of the mantra, its vibrational offerings are flowing and, like a radio station transmitting a bit further down the dial from where we're currently listening, in time we'll be able to tune in to the new frequency.

In my case, I was three or four days into the practice when I felt that I was finally able to begin to really tune in to that energetic station of the *Maha Vidya*. The sounds of the mantra, which had previously felt awkward and unfamiliar, began to flow in a graceful stream. I found that I wasn't relying on the printed form of the mantra as much and that most of the time now I could call it forth from memory. As the practice opened itself to me more and more, I turned my attention to cultivating the feeling-tone of my intention through the practice. I began to seek my inner Saraswati.

As I sat every day for the *Maha Vidya* practice, I would use my breath to amp up my inner experience of the mantra's vibrations.

In particular, engaging ujjayi breath noticeably fanned the flames of the subtler resonance of the mantra inside. As the resonance and energies of the mantra began to build within me during the practice, I turned my heart and mind toward the radiant, living energies and qualities of Saraswati, the embodiment of Divinely-inspired creative artistry.

I'd often begin this aspect of the practice with visualization, calling to mind as vividly as I could the vibrant image of Saraswati. I'll be the first to admit, I'm not really that adept in the art of visualization, but even so, I was still able to imagine the broad strokes of Saraswati's iconography: sitting atop a blooming white lotus, a flowing river behind her, a *vina* (ancient Indian lute) resting on her lap, a japa mala in one hand, a sacred scripture emanating wisdom in the other. These details were peripheral to me, though, compared to her most clearly defined feature: her loving gaze. It's a look that conveys infinite love and beneficence; it's a look that says, *All is well. You've got this. The creative energy of the Universe is flowing through your heart and mind this very moment.*

As my daily mantra practice unfolded, I would return again and again to Saraswati's loving gaze within my mind's eye and I would savor the palpable feelings those beneficent eyes conveyed. Those feelings of love, openness, and joy would permeate me as I then began to imagine this Divine creative energy manifesting itself in my own life. I would imagine myself sitting at the computer, words flowing freely and joyfully from my mind and heart. I would see myself happily completing my work on the book day after day, and I would allow myself to feel exactly what I would feel *as if this were actually happening right here and now.* Other times, when I found it difficult to imagine myself in this abundance of creative flow, I'd pray with deep humility and love, asking

Spirit to guide me and fill me with all I'd need to complete this work for the highest good of myself, my family, my community, and my world.

Utilizing my breath as a kind of pranic or energetic thread, I would string together one glimpse, one experience, one *darshan* after another. By the end of the mantra practice, I would find that this succession of energetic, felt emotional experiences had threaded together to make a kind of vibrational garland—an internal, energetic mala that had now become a part of my being. All the while, the healing vibrations of the *Maha Vidya* mantra reverberated within me, purifying me and aligning me with the energies of my highest intentions.

As I write these words, I'm completing the final week of my 40-day Saraswati mantra practice. The book you're now holding in your hands is proof of the power and efficacy of this practice. On so many levels, investing in ourselves through a deep practice like an anusthan—dedicating ourselves to a daily immersion in the energies, qualities, and feeling-tones of our highest ideals—is a gift of immeasurable value. At its core, it's a way of expanding beyond a limited sense of self into connection with a higher power. There's freedom and grace in that connection. And there's peace of mind in knowing that our lives are part of a greater whole.

Creating Your Own 40-Day Anusthan

As you set out to begin your own anusthan practice, take a moment to think about the most essential, important intention or issue in your life right now. What is it that you'd most like to dedicate this powerful mantra practice to healing, inspiring, transforming, releasing, or manifesting? Allow yourself the time and meditative space to receive the clearest, truest answer to this question.

Once you're clear on the intention behind your practice, you might find that a certain Deity or mantra that you discovered earlier in the Songbook for the Soul comes to mind. If not, you might have a look through the chapters of that section again while gently and mindfully holding the thought of your intention. Let your heart be your guide as you look for the mantra that feels right for you.

When you feel like you've found the perfect mantra, take some time to get familiar with the pronunciation by listening to the audio link of your chosen mantra. Get acquainted with the sounds of the mantra before beginning your anusthan. You'll also want to experiment with doing japa of your mantra to see exactly how many rounds you intend to complete for your daily anusthan practice, depending on how much time you can commit to. You want to strike a balance between enough rounds to allow you to really immerse in the experience, but not so many that you might have trouble maintaining the practice over the course of forty days. You also might choose to do your anusthan at the same time every day, setting up a powerful energetic rhythm for your practice.

At the beginning of your anusthan, you can choose to set an intention for your practice, called a *sankalpa*. This is simply a heartfelt statement of your deepest intentions for doing this particular mantra practice and may be spoken out loud, said silently in your own mind and heart, or written down on a piece of paper and placed upon your altar or in a place that is special to you. Traditionally, you would offer this sankalpa on the first day of your anusthan; however, if at any time during the forty days of your practice you'd like to reaffirm or reconnect with your intention, feel free to offer it again. Also, you may want to choose to start your anusthan on an auspicious day—a full moon or a new moon, for example—or any day that feels somehow meaningful for you.

Feeling the Bhav:
Embodying Your Intentions

Now that you're ready to begin your anusthan, remember that you can enrich and enhance your daily practice with the insights and tools we've explored together in this book. Though we all come to this practice with our own unique intentions, inspiring us to embrace a wide variety of mantras, we can all deepen and enliven our experience by utilizing these same basic principles.

First, you might choose to begin your daily anusthan practice with some mindful singing. This can be as simple as singing a few *Oms*, accompanied by the sound of the tamboura drone in the musical key aligned with your vocal sweet spot. Or, perhaps before beginning the japa practice of your anusthan mantra you might choose to sing it out loud first, attuning your body and mind to the vibrations of the mantra. As you sing, remember to engage your inner flowerpot, supporting the flower of your voice as you chant the mantra. With every inhalation, feel yourself being filled with the supportive, nurturing energy of the Universe. Through mindful singing, you become more fully embodied, present, and ready to receive all the benefits of your mantra practice. Feel free to sing until your body and mind feel calm and aligned.

Once you're ready to begin your japa practice, spend the first few minutes simply tuning in to the sound vibrations of your chosen mantra within you. You might find it inspiring to have the tamboura drone playing gently in the background, providing a sweet sonic space within which your heart and mind can open. Use ujjayi breath to amplify and enhance the resonance of the mantra within you. Allow yourself to go at your own pace, savoring each repetition of the mantra and pouring your full awareness into subtle sound vibrations inside.

When you feel that your mantra is flowing naturally and easily, begin to invite the feeling-tone of your intention into the practice. Through visualization and contemplation, bring forth the feelings and energetic qualities of your intention—making them as real and palpable as you possibly can—while continuing to immerse yourself in the repetition of your mantra. See and imagine yourself experiencing the complete realization of your intentions. Allow yourself to feel this with every cell of your being. Breathe it in as you continue to immerse yourself in the healing vibrations of your mantra.

Once you've completed your practice, give yourself a few minutes to absorb the energies you've generated. You might choose to do a few rounds of alternate nostril breathing (nadi shodhana) to deeply align with the energetic qualities of your practice. When you're ready for your mantra practice to come to a close, you might choose to place both hands on your heart, knowing that the healing energies you've cultivated will continue to resonate within you. As you go about your day, you can take a moment to silently repeat your mantra to yourself, affirming the intentions of your practice anytime you choose.

On the last day of your 40-day anusthan, take a moment and return to the intention that inspired you to take up this practice, your sankalpa. If you've chosen to write your intention down on a piece of paper, you might take it out and look at it. As you think about the intention that brought you to this practice, notice what shifts and changes may have taken place in your life over these past forty days. For some of us, those changes may be profound and dramatic—outwardly manifesting for all to see. For others, those changes may happen more subtly, with the inner transformation of our perception and understanding.

Take a moment to notice these changes in your life and to express gratitude that you've chosen to invest in your happiness and well-being by embracing these healing practices. Know that your heart and your voice harmonize with those of millions of other beautiful souls all around the world, joining together in this global choir of mindful singing, music, and mantra.

Acknowledgments

This book would not have been possible without the constant love and support of my wife, Virginia, who knew and believed that I could bring forth this creative offering even before I did. I want to express my tremendous gratitude to Zhena Muzyka and Enliven Books for the invitation and the support to bring this vision into reality. Zhena has been connected to my music from the very beginning and it's incredibly gratifying to collaborate with her on this next evolutionary leap. Thank you for giving me the opportunity to take the writer's journey of self-discovery. I also want to offer my heartfelt thanks to Emily Han at Lyrical Editing for her clarity, insight, and support in making this book the best that it could be. And a special thanks to my mom and dad, who started it all with that little red snare drum back when I was eight years old and have supported my musical dreams from day one.

I also want to offer my profound gratitude for the wise and loving guidance of my teachers, Shankaracharya Swami and Babaji Bob Kindler, who embody the grace and blessings of living a Divine life. Special thanks to Shankaracharya Swami for graciously contributing his translations for several of the chants and hymns in the Songbook for the Soul. I also want to thank my old friend Krishna Das for generously contributing his translation of the *Hanuman Chalisa* to the book. Sitting beside him on my tablas back in 1999, he showed me what it was like to bring the ashram out into the world. Many thanks as well to Swami Satyananda Saraswati for his lovely translation of the *Devi Suktam* chant. I'm also deeply grateful to Rajeshwari Gretchen Carmel for contributing her beautiful insights and translations for the japa mantras in the back of the book.

All of the stunning and inspiring artwork in *Music and Mantras* was created by my friend Paul Heussenstamm, who came to my very first public kirtan in Joshua Tree, California, back in 2005. For more than ten years, I've been a huge fan of Paul's painting and to be able share his radiant, enchanting visions with you all here is a dream come true. Thank you, Paul!

The sweet sounds of the mantra recordings that grace this book were produced in collaboration with my friend and audio guru, Hans Christian. For more than a decade, I've turned to Hans when it was time to share my music with the world. His sonic artistry and the sweet sounds of his cello and sarangi truly bring the soundtrack of *Music and Mantras* to a whole new level. Thank you, Hans.

I'd also like to express my heartfelt gratitude to Daniel Comstock from the Center for Attitudinal Healing & the Arts for his invaluable insights about the yoga of mindful singing. Daniel's wisdom and insights about music and singing opened my eyes to an even greater depth of appreciation for the healing power the human voice. Many thanks as well to the amazing Kate Hart from the Holistic Voice Institute, who brought some Detroit soul into the mix and shared her fabulous vocal tips with me.

The wealth of scientific research studies cited in the book were generously provided to me by Steve Farmer, PhD, whose passion for discovering and sharing modern scientific insights about the ancient practice of yoga has been a great inspiration.

I want to give a shout-out to my brothers and sisters in the kirtan world, circling the globe with me to share the joy of music and chanting: David Newman, Sean Johnson and The Wild Lotus Band, Donna De Lory, Dave Stringer, Wah, Snatam Kaur, Jai Uttal, Krishna Das, Deva Premal & Miten, GuruGanesha, Shantala, and so many more. It's an honor to share this journey with you.

Over the yearlong adventure of writing this book, I had the great fortune to call upon the insight and support of my friends Rolf and Mariam Gates, who were a tremendous source of inspiration and guidance along the way. Thank you!

Finally, I want to thank my daughters, Hannah and Tara, for bringing so much love and joy into my life. May this book bring a little more light and peace into the world that awaits you.

GIRISH
MARCH 9, 2016
SANTA CRUZ, CA

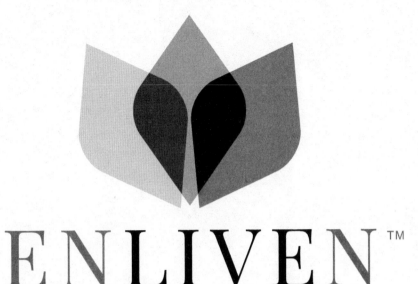

ENLIVEN™

About Our Books: We are the world's first holistic publisher for mission-driven authors. We curate, create, collaborate on, and commission sophisticated, fresh titles and voices to enhance your spiritual development, success, and wellness pursuits.

About Our Vision: Our authors are the voice of empowerment, creativity, and spirituality in the twenty-first century. You, our readers, are brilliant seekers of adventure, unexpected stories, and tools to transform yourselves and your world. Together, we are change-makers on a mission to increase literacy, uplift humanity, ignite genius, and create reasons to gather around books. We think of ourselves as instigators of soulful exchange.

Enliven Books is a new imprint from social entrepreneur and publisher Zhena Muzyka, author of *Life by the Cup.*

To explore our list of books and learn about fresh new voices in the realm of Mind-Body-Spirit, please visit us at

EnlivenBooks.com | **/EnlivenBooks**

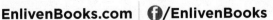

A Note on the Harmonium

It's easy to play any musical instrument: all you have
to do is touch the right key at the right time and the
instrument will play itself.

—Johann Sebastian Bach

In my travels around the country, in nearly every city in which I
have the good fortune to sing, at least one person will approach
me after the chant and ask, "What *is* this instrument?" pointing
to my harmonium with a quizzical but bliss-filled expression. "It's
a meditation machine," I like to say, and that explanation seems to
suit everyone just fine.

Of course, I'll also share what I know about the harmonium
as a musical instrument, where it came from and how it works.
But the thing about the harmonium is that *sound*. Those sweet,
rich tones are so undeniably intoxicating. I like to invite people
try it for themselves, to show them how easy it is to hold down a
couple of notes with one hand and gently pump the bellows with
the other. The harmonium has a way of playing *through* you. It fills
you up, like a third lung, lifting and strengthening your voice. So,
if you've always loved the sound of the harmonium but have never
taken, say, a BINA 23 B Deluxe for a spin yourself, then you're in
for a whole new experience entirely.

A Little History

The search for an instrument that could produce precisely this kind of intoxicating sound is, in fact, what led to the creation of the harmonium in the first place. Europeans in the eighteenth century were eager to find a more economical means of obtaining the coveted tones of a church organ—an instrument out of the financial reach of most musicians. (And besides, even if you could afford one, where would you *put* it?)

These eighteenth-century musical explorers found echoes of this sound in an Asian flute called the *sheng* (pronounced "shung," meaning "life" or "sublime voice"), which is thought to date back to 3000 BC or earlier. The sheng traditionally featured a cluster of seventeen bamboo pipes arranged like the two folded wings of a bird. As the player breathed in through this ancient instrument (rather than blowing out), the metal or bamboo reeds within each pipe would vibrate to produce the sheng's haunting, resonant tone. This instrument, or one of its later incarnations, eventually made its way west sometime around the early seventeenth century and caught the ears of savvy European musicians. These instruments, though primitive, actually form the roots of the harmonium's family tree and produce their sound in basically the same way.

The "Free-Reed" Family

The harmonium, accordion, harmonica, and concertina are all part of the "free-reed" family and inherit their unique sound from their ancient Chinese ancestors. All of these instruments create sound by vibrating one end of a thin reed, while the other end is held stationary. To see the free-reed effect in action, find yourself a thin plastic ruler and a table or desk. While holding one end of the ruler down firmly with your palm, allow four to five inches to extend out over the edge of the table. Now, pluck the free end of the ruler with your finger and, voilà! You can experiment with changing the tone by changing how much you allow to hang over the edge.

You can chart the evolution of the free-reed instruments from the *naw* (the likely grandfather of the sheng that featured bamboo reeds attached to two pipes mounted on a gourd) all the way up to the modern harmonium (which boasts nearly one hundred metal reeds, a two-and-a-half- to three-and-a-half-octave keyboard, a bellows to supply the air, and air stop knobs to open different reed chambers—all easily collapsible into a portable little package which fits quite nicely into the overhead bin of a plane).

It was Alexandre Debain, a Frenchman, who invented the first actual harmonium in 1842. His invention, and many others that followed during the harmonium's first heyday in the nineteenth century, would have been hardly recognizable to fans of the modern harmonium. These large, ornate instruments were played while sitting in a chair and using foot pedals to pump the air. They became very popular in Victorian homes during a time when church hymns were typical fare in drawing-room music.

It wasn't until 1875 that an Indian, Dwarkanath Ghose, simplified Debain's design and created a harmonium meant to be played while seated on the floor. Mr. Ghose's innovation also introduced the hand bellows, leaving just one hand free to play the keyboard. This was a unique reflection of the Indian musical sensibility, which emphasizes melody rather than chords. It's Ghose's design that has persisted and flourished to this day.

Resources

The harmonium is alive and well in the twenty-first century, perhaps more so now than ever before. It's an instrument that is easily accessible, fairly easy to play, and a great asset to chanting practice. If you're inspired to pick up a harmonium for yourself, you'll find a few of my favorite instrument shops listed in the Recommended Resources Guide.

Recommended Resources Guide

Harmoniums and Tambouras

Musician's Mall

Based in Berkeley, CA, Musicians's Mall (formerly the Ali Akbar College of Music Store) has a wide variety of high-quality Indian musical instruments including harmoniums, tambouras, tablas, and more.
www.MusiciansMallUSA.com
1-510-225-9597

Keshav Music Imports

If you happen to be harmonium shopping on the East Coast, you might want to check out New York's Keshav Music Imports. They feature hand-selected harmoniums, tambouras, tablas, and more.
www.Keshav-Music.com
1-212-228-7864

India Abundance

India Abundance is a new online resource that offers harmoniums and much more shipped directly from India. They offer speedy global shipping and the lowest prices I've found for harmoniums.

www.IndiaAbundance.com

+91-11-42381038

Japa Malas

Yoga Basics

At the Yoga Basics website, you'll find a variety of beautiful malas made with semiprecious gemstones, hand-carved bone, rudraksha beads, sacred woods, and hemp tassels.

www.yogabasics.com

Mala for Vets

Mala for Vets is a Baltimore-based veteran-owned and veteran-made mala resource that donates its proceeds to provide yoga for veterans. You'll find a wide selection of malas here, including a series made from gemstones associated with the various chakras.

www.malaforvets.org

Buddha Groove

This site offers a nice selection of affordable malas, including ones made from rudraksha seeds, sandalwood, and gemstones.

www.buddhagroove.com/meditation-mala

Nectar

The Nectar website offers many different mala styles including rudraksha, gemstones, and woods, and uses their

proceeds to fund projects benefitting immigrant, at-risk, and refugee youth, both locally and globally.
www.shop.amalafoundation.org/default.asp

Karmic Jewels By Nadine

This site offers gorgeous, high-end malas made of semiprecious gemstones—some of which feature beautiful images of various Deities. Proceeds from all sales through Karmic Jewels go to benefit the victims of sex trafficking in India.
www.karmicjewelsbynadine.com

Satya Jewelry

Satya Scainetti's beautiful and empowering malas feature semi-precious gemstones revered for their ancient healing properties. Sales from her site support a variety of wonderful charities benefiting Indian women and children.
www.satyajewelry.com

Books

Mantra Resources:

Healing Mantras by Thomas Ashley-Farrand (Random House Publishing Group, 1999)

Shakti Mantras by Thomas Ashley-Farrand (Random House Publishing Group, 2003)

Chakra Mantras by Thomas Ashley-Farrand (Red Wheel/Weiser, 2006)

Mantra Yoga & Primal Sound by Dr. David Frawley (Lotus Press, 2010)

Tools for Tantra by Harish Johari (Destiny Books, 1988)

The Nectar of Chanting by Swami Muktananda and Bhagavan Nityananda (Syda Foundation, 1984)

The World Is Sound: Nada Brahma by Joachim-Ernst Berendt (Destiny Books, 1991)

Words of Wisdom from the Saints:

Great Swan: Meetings with Ramakrishna by Lex Hixon (Larson Publications, 1997)

Coming Home: The Experience of Enlightenment in Sacred Traditions by Lex Hixon (Larson Publications, 1995)

Karma-Yoga and Bhakti-Yoga by Swami Vivekananda (Ramakrishna Vivekananda Center, 1982)

Raja-Yoga by Swami Vivekananda (Ramakrishna Vivekananda Center, 1982)

Jnana-Yoga by Swami Vivekananda (Ramakrishna Vivekananda Center, 1982)

The Upanishads translations by Eknath Easwaran (Nilgiri Press, 1987)

The Essential Teachings of Ramana Maharshi by Ramana Maharshi (Inner Directions Publishing, 2001)

Autobiography of a Yogi by Paramahansa Yogananda (Self-Realization Fellowship, 1977)

Journey of Awakening by Ram Dass (Bantam, 1990)

Neuroscience and the New Biology:

Buddha's Brain by Rick Hanson, PhD (New Harbinger Publications, 2009)

Hardwiring Happiness by Rick Hanson, PhD (Harmony Books, 2013)

The Brain that Changes Itself by Norman Doidge (Penguin Books, 2007)

This Is Your Brain on Music by Daniel J. Levitin (Plume/Penguin, 2007)

The World in Six Songs by Daniel J. Levitin (Dutton, 2009)

The Biology of Belief by Bruce Lipton (Hay House, 2008)

Spontaneous Evolution: Our Positive Future (and a Way to Get There From Here) by Bruce Lipton and Steve Bhaerman (Hay House, 2010)

Mantra Music

Spirit Voyage
You'll find a wide variety of mantra and chanting music here, with an emphasis on chants from the Kundalini Yoga tradition. www.spiritvoyage.com

White Swan Music
White Swan offers an immense selection of mantra, chanting, and yoga-related music to choose from. www.whiteswanmusic.com

All Things Girish

At the Girish Music website, you'll find a complete listing of Girish's tour dates, chanting events, and retreats; Girish CDs, DVDs, and music downloads; as well as booking information if you'd like to arrange an event in your area.
www.girishmusic.com

Glossary

Ajapa Japa: Constant internal repetition of a mantra, often connected with the natural flow of the breath, without the aid of a mala.

Ajna: The 6th Chakra (energy center), or Third Eye, located between the eyebrows and associated with wisdom and insight.

Anahata: The 4th Chakra (energy center), located at the heart and associated with love, empathy, and balance between masculine and feminine energies.

Anahata Nada: The name Anahata comes from a Sanskrit word that literally means "unstruck," referring to the "unstruck sound," deep reverberations of the inner *Om* experienced in the heart.

Anusthan: A dedicated period of mantra practice, often for forty days, undertaken for a particular intention.

Asana: The physical postures of Hatha Yoga, designed to cultivate ease, balance, and relaxation in the body, preparing the way for concentration and meditation.

Ashram: A spiritual center or yogic hermitage, often the abode of a Guru or living master with whom students come to learn.

Bhakti Yoga: A path of yoga emphasizing direct experience of the Divine through mantra, chanting, and other devotional practices. The Bhakti movement originated in seventh-century India and espoused the universal nature of spirituality available to all and everyone through direct experience, rejecting traditional divisions of caste and creed.

Bhava: A deep and absorbing experience, associated with exalted and blissful states cultivated through yogic practices such as mantra and meditation. From the Sanskrit, meaning "state of existence."

Bija: A single-syllable mantra, or primal "seed sound," such as *Om*. Bija mantras are considered to be powerful distillations of pure mantra sound vibration and, as such, are not translatable.

Chakras: The seven major energy centers of the human body identified by the yogic tradition, beginning at the base of the spine and ascending up to the crown of the head. Each chakra is said to have its own sound (bija), energetic quality, and color. The word *chakra* means "wheel" or "circle" in Sanskrit.

Chi: A Chinese word signifying life force or energy flow, similar to the yogic term *prana*.

Dan Tien: The center of our physical and energetic bodies, located one and one-half thumb widths below the navel and two to three thumb widths inside the body.

Darshan: The vision of a Deity experienced within. Sometimes refers to being in the presence of a saint or holy person. From the Sanskrit, meaning "to see."

Devanagari: The ancient alphabet of the Sanskrit language, which consists of forty-seven characters—fourteen vowels and thirty-three consonants. The *Om* symbol is a familiar example of the Devanagari script.

Dharma: In Hinduism, this word implies "right action" or "right livelihood," while in Buddhism it refers to the teachings of the Buddha and the idea of "universal truth" or "cosmic order."

Durga: The Hindu goddess who embodies the energies and powers of all the gods. She represents Shakti, the grace-bestowing feminine principle that guides us from lifetime to lifetime. The Sanskrit word *durga* literally means "difficult," and She is known as the Remover of Difficulties.

Ganesh (also Ganapati): The elephant-headed Deity who represents the primal root energy of consciousness. Known as the Remover of Obstacles, Ganesh embodies the unity of all life and existence.

Hanuman: The Hindu Deity who embodies supreme selfless devotion, strength, courage, humility, and awakened prana—the powerful spiritual vitality that arises from a life lived in service to a higher ideal. As the foremost devotee of Lord Rama, Hanuman's exploits are told in the famous Hindu epic the *Ramayana*.

Harmonium: The Indian reed organ often used in kirtan and other forms of devotional chanting. This instrument produces sound when air from the bellows vibrates a series of thin metal reeds, much like an accordion.

Japa: The repetition of mantra with the aid of a mala. The mantra may be recited either softly or purely within the mind and heart of the meditator.

Jnana Yoga: The yogic path of spiritual union through wisdom or knowledge. One of the four classic paths of yoga, the other three being Karma Yoga (the path of selfless action or service), Bhakti Yoga (the path of love and devotion), and Raja Yoga (the path of meditation).

Kirtan: A form of devotional call-and-response chanting of the "names of God" in which the kirtan leader sings out a particular mantra and the group sings it back in response.

Krishna: The Hindu Deity embodying the ideal of pure, ecstatic love. The tales and teachings of Krishna figure prominently in the *Bhagavad Gita*, a part of the great Hindu epic the *Mahabharata*.

Kundalini: The primal, spiritual energy that lies coiled at the base of the spine. The practices of yoga are intended to awaken this dormant energy, causing it to ascend up through the energy centers of the chakras, purifying them, and culminating in Self-realization or enlightenment.

Lakshmi: The Hindu goddess who embodies the auspicious qualities of prosperity, royal power, success, and illustriousness. She represents not only financial abundance, but an abundance of anything we value in life: love, good health, harmonious relationships, peace, and more.

Likhita Japa: The writing out of mantras by hand, either upon the image of a Deity or simply line by line. This form of mantra practice is said to be particularly engaging, inspiring a deep harmony between the mind and the heart.

Lila: Pronounced "Leela," this Sanskrit word means "play" or "sport." It conveys the notion that all of life is the joyful dance of the Divine, blissfully sporting with itself through all names and forms.

Mala: Prayer beads that are used for japa mantra practice. There are 108 beads on a mala, with one extra "guru" or "meru" bead that signifies the start and end point of the round. Traditionally held in the right hand, the beads of the mala pass between the thumb and the middle finger with each repetition of the mantra.

Manipura: The 3rd Chakra (energy center), located at the navel center and associated with self-esteem and willpower.

Mantra: Translated literally as "mind tool" or "mind liberator," a mantra is a sound vibration—chanted out loud or internally—through which we mindfully focus our thoughts, our feelings, and our highest intentions.

Meru: The 109th bead on a mala (rosary) that serves to mark the start and end point of one round of japa practice. Traditionally, when one reaches the meru bead, one reverses direction and begins the next round of japa anew, rather than crossing over the meru bead. The Sanskrit word *meru* literally means "mountain."

Mudra: From the Sanskrit word meaning "gesture" or "seal," a mudra is a yogic hand gesture that is said to connect certain energy meridians, guiding and directing energies in the body and mind. A mudra can be seen as an outer manifestation of our internal thoughts and prayers, amplifying and expressing our intentions.

Muladhara: The 1st Chakra (energy center), located at the base of the spine and associated with the grounding energy of the earth, security, and fulfilling material needs.

Murti: An image or statue of a Deity. In the Hindu tradition, a murti is not thought of as an idol but, rather, as a Divine image that brings to mind the reality of the beloved in the same way that a photograph of someone we love brings the presence of that person to our minds and hearts.

Nadi Shodhana: Alternate nostril pranayama, or yogic breathing, the name of which means "clearing the channels of circulation." Using the right hand to block one nostril and then the other, even and alternating breaths are taken through the left and right nostrils, bringing balance and calm to the body and mind.

Prana: The vital life force that exists in all of creation. This revitalizing and healing energy can be cultivated through the practices of yoga, mantra, chanting, and pranayama.

Pranayama: Yogic breathing techniques that use alternate nostril breathing, retention, *bandhas* (energy locks), and a variety of other breathing methods to cultivate greater balance, vitality, mental clarity, and concentration.

Raga: The musical system of melodic modes used in Indian classical music. The word *raga* literally means "color" or "hue," implying how these various musical modes influence or color the listener's emotions, mood, and energy. A raga is not merely a musical scale but rather an intricate combination of scale, dominant notes, ascending and descending lines, musical ornaments, and more; each of which is associated with a particular mood, time of day, and season.

Rudraksha: The seeds that are produced by a particular evergreen tree that is native to northern India as well as several other countries. Since at least the tenth century, yogis in the Hindu and Buddhist traditions have sought these seeds in order to make japa malas from them. Rudraksha malas are believed to aid in accumulating the beneficial energy generated through mantra practice, to protect the wearer against negativity, and are said to have healing properties.

Sadhana: Any kind of yogic practice, such as mantra, meditation, pranayama, study of the scriptures, pilgrimage, etc., undertaken for the purpose of advancing on the spiritual path.

Sahasrara: The 7th Chakra (energy center), or Thousand-petaled Lotus, located at the crown of the head and associated with blissful union, transcendence of individuality, and self-realization.

Samskaras: The deep mental or psychological tendencies that build up through the repetition of particular actions, thoughts, and feelings, creating a kind of energetic impression. These samskaras are thought to be at the root of habitual thought and behavior. One can dissolve these limiting karmic patterns through the practices of yoga.

Sankalpa: A one-pointed and heartfelt resolve that is stated at the beginning of a significant undertaking, such as a mantra anusthan, expressing the highest intention of the practitioner.

Saraswati: The Hindu goddess of music, arts, learning, wisdom, and creative flow. She is said to be the one who leads to the essence of self-knowledge.

Sargam: The syllables associated with the seven notes of the musical scale in the Indian classical tradition (*Sa, Re, Ga, Ma, Pa, Dha,* and *Ni*).

Sarod: A fretless, lute-like stringed instrument that is one of the most widely known in the Indian music tradition, made popular around the world by Ali Akbar Khan.

Seva: The act of selfless service as a kind of spiritual practice. This is Karma Yoga in action—acting for the benefit of others with a sense of gratitude and openhearted kindness.

Shakti: The universal Divine feminine principle that is the creative, dynamic energy of consciousness. In the Tantric worldview, Shakti is the revealing, grace-bestowing energy that awakens us to our higher spiritual nature.

Shiva: The Hindu Deity who represents both the Divine archetype of pure wisdom beyond any trace of illusion as well as the embodiment of the original yogi, meditating in the exalted, snowy peaks of Mount Kailash in the Himalayas. In the Tantric worldview, Shiva is the universal Divine masculine principle that is the static, transcendent reality underlying all existence.

Sitar: A large classical Indian stringed instrument, made popular by Ravi Shankar, with a distinctive, resonant sound that is instantly recognizable. It's believed to have evolved from an ancient Indian instrument called the vina.

Svadhisthana: The 2nd Chakra (energy center), or Sacral Center, located about two fingers' width below the navel and associated with creativity, sexuality, connection, and relationship.

Tabla: The hand drums of classical Indian music, comprised of a higher-pitched wooden drum (*dayan*) and a lower-pitched metal drum (*bayan*).

Tala: The rhythmic patterns of Indian music, which refer to the number of beats per measure as well as the emphasis and groupings of those beats.

Tamboura (also Tanpura or Tambura): An Indian stringed instrument resembling a large lute, used for producing drones for musical accompaniment.

Ujjayi: The "ocean sounding breath" that is used in many yogic practices, produced by gently constricting the opening in the back of the throat while breathing in and out through the nose. (This is the same effect produced naturally when we whisper.) Ujjayi lengthens and deepens the breath, enhances concentration, warms the core of the body by warming the incoming air, and strengthens the nervous and digestive systems.

Vishuddha: The 5th Chakra (energy center), located in the area of the throat and associated with self-expression and communication.

Wallah: A Hindi word meaning "someone who performs a certain service," as in, "We got a cup of tea from the chai wallah." The word is sometimes used to describe someone who leads chanting as a "kirtan wallah."

Notes

1. Daniel Comstock (Director for the Center for Attitudinal Healing & the Arts), in discussion with the author, December 2015.
2. Daniel J. Levitin, *This Is Your Brain on Music: The Science of a Human Obsession* (New York: Penguin Group, 2006), 153–54.
3. Sarah C. P. Williams, "Singing Kick Starts Social Bonding," *Science Magazine* (October 27, 2015), http://www.sciencemag.org/news/2015/10/singing-kick-starts-social-bonding.
4. Christina Grape et al., "Does Singing Promote Well-Being?: An Empirical Study of Professional and Amateur Singers During a Singing Lesson," *Integrative Physiological & Behavioral Science* 38, no.1 (January–March 2003): 65–74.
5. HeartMath Institute, "Heart Rate Variability," October 27, 2014, https://www.heartmath.org/articles-of-the-heart/the-math-of-heartmath/heart-rate-variability/#more-5640.
6. Björn Vickhoff et al., "Music Structure Determines Heart Rate Variability of Singers," *Frontiers in Psychology* (July 9, 2013): http://dx.doi.org/10.3389/fpsyg.2013.00334.
7. Luciano Bernardi et al., "Effect of Rosary Prayer and Yoga Mantras On Autonomic Cardiovascular Rhythms," *British Medical Journal* 323, no. 7327 (December 22–29, 2001).
8. Gene D. Cohen, MD, PhD, "The Creativity and Aging Study," National Endowments for the Arts and George Washington University, April 2006.
9. Ibid.
10. J. K. Johnson et al., "Quality of Life (QOL) of Older Adult Community

Choral Singers in Finland," *International Psychogeriatrics* 25, no. 7 (July 2013): 1–10, http://www.ncbi.nlm.nih.gov/pubmed/23574947.

11. Stacy Horn, "Singing Changes Your Brain," *Time*, August 16, 2013.

12. Daniel Comstock (Director for the Center for Attitudinal Healing & the Arts), in discussion with the author, December 2015.

13. Kate Hart (Director of the Holistic Voice Institute and Michigan Voice Over Talent), in discussion with the author, November 2015.

14. Norman Doidge, MD, *The Brain That Changes Itself: Stories of Personal Triumph from the Frontiers of Brain Science* (New York: Penguin Books, 2007), 9.

15. "How to Become Batman," *Invisibilia*, podcast audio, January 23, 2015.

16. Lore Thaler, Stephen R. Arnott, and Melvyn A. Goodale, "Human Echolocation I," *Journal of Vision* 10 (August 2010): 1050.

17. Carla Shatz, "The Developing Brain," *Scientific American* 267, no. 3 (September 1992): 60–67.

18. Rick Hanson, PhD, *Hardwiring Happiness: The New Brain Science of Contentment, Calm, and Confidence* (New York: Harmony Books, 2013), 15.

19. Ibid., 14.

20. Christian Gaser and Gottfried Schlaug, "Brain Structures Differ between Musicians and Non-Musicians," *The Journal of Neuroscience* 23, no. 27 (October 8, 2003): 9240–45.

21. Sue McGreevey, "Eight Weeks to a Better Brain," *Harvard Gazette*, January 21, 2011, http://news.harvard.edu/gazette/story/2011/01/eight-weeks-to-a-better-brain.

22. Hanson, *Hardwiring Happiness*, 60.

23. Ibid., 119.

24. Paramahansa Yogananda, *Autobiography of a Yogi* (Los Angeles: Self-Realization Fellowship, 1946).

25. Hanson, *Hardwiring Happiness*, 15.

26. *The Upanishads*, trans. Juan Mascaró (London: Penguin Classics, 1965), 7.

27. Ibid., 83.

28. Father Steven Peter Tsichlis, "The Jesus Prayer," *Greek Orthodox Archdiocese of America*, http://www.goarch.org/ourfaith/ourfaith7104.

29. Ganesh mantra translations written in collaboration with Rajeshwari

Gretchen Carmel, owner/director: the Yoga Space (Keene, NH), certified Sanskrit mantra teacher and ordained Pujari/Vedic priest in Sanatana Dharma Satsang by Namadeva Acharya (Thomas Ashley-Farrand).

30. Lakshmi mantra translations written in collaboration with Rajeshwari Gretchen Carmel.

31. *Mahaalakshmyashtakam*, trans. by Shankaracharya Swami, *Sacred Hymns* (Boulder: Sadhana Ashram, Inc., 2002), 42.

32. Hanuman mantra translations written in collaboration with Rajeshwari Gretchen Carmel.

33. *Hanuman Chalisa*, trans. by Krishna Das, used with permission, www .KrishnaDas.com.

34. Lex Hixon, *Mother of the Universe* (Wheaton, IL: Quest Books, 1994), 46.

35. Shakti mantra translations written in collaboration with Rajeshwari Gretchen Carmel.

36. *Devi Suktam*, trans. by Swami Satyananda Saraswati, *Chandi Path* (Delhi: Devi Mandir Publications and Motilal Banarsidass Publishers, 1995), 348–56.

37. *Shri Devi Ashtottara*, trans. by Shankaracharya Swami, *Sacred Hymns*, 32–38.

38. Shiva mantra translations written in collaboration with Rajeshwari Gretchen Carmel.

39. *Nirvanashatkam*, trans. by Shankaracharya Swami, *Sacred Chants*, 57–58, with contributions from Swami Jnaneshvara Bharati.

40. Mantra translations written in collaboration with Rajeshwari Gretchen Carmel.

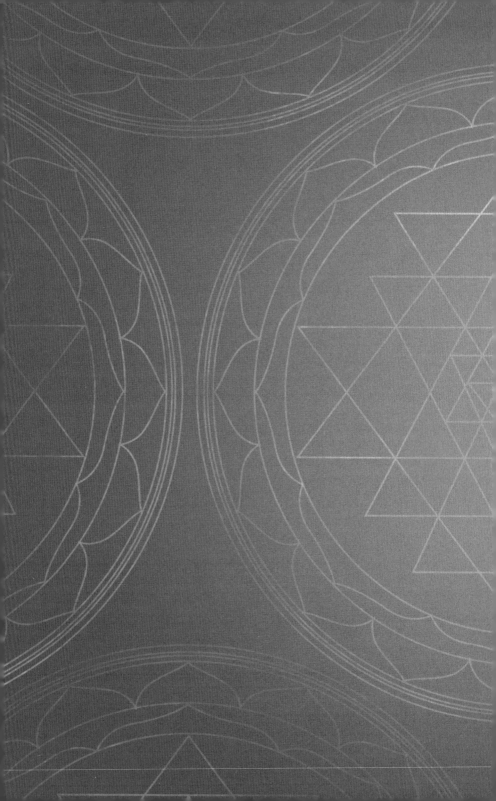